SOAP
for
Neurology

Check out the entire SOAP series!

SOAP for Cardiology
SOAP for Emergency Medicine
SOAP for Family Medicine
SOAP for Internal Medicine
SOAP for Obstetrics and Gynecology
SOAP for Neurology
SOAP for Orthopedics
SOAP for Pediatrics
SOAP for Urology

SOAP for Neurology

Frank P. Lin, MD
Clinical Neurophysiology Fellow
University of Southern California Keck School of Medicine
Los Angeles, California

Series Editor
Peter S. Uzelac, MD, FACOG
Assistant Professor
Department of Obstetrics and Gynecology
University of Southern California Keck School of Medicine
Los Angeles, California

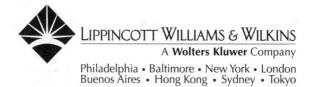

LIPPINCOTT WILLIAMS & WILKINS
A **Wolters Kluwer** Company
Philadelphia • Baltimore • New York • London
Buenos Aires • Hong Kong • Sydney • Tokyo

Acquisitions Editor: Beverly Copland
Development Editor: Selene Steneck
Production Editor: Jennifer Kowalewski
Interior and Cover Designer: Meral Dabcovich
Compositor: International Typesetting and Composition in India
Printer: Sheridan Books in Ann Arbor, MI

Copyright © 2006 Frank P. Lin, MD

351 West Camden Street
Baltimore, MD 21201

530 Walnut Street
Philadelphia, PA 19106

All rights reserved. This book is protected by copyright. No part of this book may be reproduced in any form or by any means, including photocopying, or utilized by any information storage and retrieval system without written permission from the copyright owner.

The publisher is not responsible (as a matter of product liability, negligence, or otherwise) for any injury resulting from any material contained herein. This publication contains information relating to general principles of medical care that should not be construed as specific instructions for individual patients. Manufacturers' product information and package inserts should be reviewed for current information, including contraindications, dosages, and precautions.

Printed in the United States of America

Library of Congress Cataloging-in-Publication Data

Lin, Frank P.
 SOAP for neurology / [edited by] Frank P. Lin.
   p. ; cm. — (SOAP series)
 Includes index.
 ISBN-13: 978-1-4051-0457-9 (pbk. : alk. paper)
 ISBN-10: 1-4051-0457-0 (pbk. : alk. paper) 1. Neurology—Handbooks, manuals, etc. 2. Neurology—Outlines, syllabi, etc.
 [DNLM: 1. Diagnostic Techniques, Neurological—Handbooks. 2. Nervous System Diseases—diagnosis—Handbooks. 3. Nervous System Diseases—therapy—Handbooks. WL 39 L735s 2006] I. Title. II. Series.

 RC343.4.L54 2006
 616.8—dc22
                          2005010319

The publishers have made every effort to trace the copyright holders for borrowed material. If they have inadvertently overlooked any, they will be pleased to make the necessary arrangements at the first opportunity.

To purchase additional copies of this book, call our customer service department at **(800) 638-3030** or fax orders to **(301) 824-7390**. International customers should call **(301) 714-2324**.

Visit Lippincott Williams & Wilkins on the Internet: http://www.LWW.com. Lippincott Williams & Wilkins customer service representatives are available from 8:30 am to 6:00 pm, EST.

Dedicated to my parents, brother, and wife

Contents

To the Reader	ix
Reviewers	x
Abbreviations	xi
Normal Lab Values	xv

I. Evaluation — 1
1. Neurologic Evaluation — 2

II. Strokes and Critical Care — 5
2. Ischemic Stroke — 6
3. Hemorrhagic Stroke — 8
4. Transient Ischemic Attack — 10
5. Cerebral Venous Thrombosis — 12
6. Strokes in Children and Young Adults — 14
7. Subarachnoid Hemorrhage — 16
8. Hydrocephalus — 18
9. Increased Intracranial Pressure — 20
10. Vascular Malformations — 22
11. Traumatic Brain Injury — 24

III. Seizures — 27
12. First Time Seizure — 28
13. Epilepsy — 30
14. Status Epilepticus — 32
15. Epilepsy Syndromes — 34
16. Localization Related Epilepsies — 36

IV. Altered Mental Status — 39
17. Altered Mental Status — 40
18. Brain Death — 42
19. Wernicke-Korsakoff Syndrome — 44

V. CNS Infectious Disease — 47
20. Bacterial Meningitis — 48
21. Herpes and Other Viral Encephalitides — 50
22. Neurosyphilis — 52
23. Neurocysticercosis — 54
24. Creutzfeldt-Jakob Disease — 56
25. Lyme Disease — 58
26. Opportunistic Infections — 60

VI. Spinal Cord Disease — 63
27. Acute Spinal Cord Syndromes — 64
28. Spasticity and Muscle Spasms — 66

VII. Neuro-Ophthalmology and Otology — 69
29. Optic Neuritis and Neuropathies — 70
30. Cavernous Sinus Syndrome — 72

31.	Diplopia	74
32.	Horner Syndrome	76
33.	Dizziness and Vertigo	78

VIII. Neuromuscular Disease — 81
- 34. Myasthenia Gravis — 82
- 35. Guillain-Barré Syndrome — 84
- 36. Botulism — 86
- 37. Peripheral Neuropathy — 88
- 38. Chronic Inflammatory Demyelinating Polyradiculoneuropathy — 90
- 39. Myopathies and Myositis — 92
- 40. Muscular Dystrophies — 94
- 41. Amyotrophic Lateral Sclerosis — 96
- 42. Entrapment Neuropathies — 98
- 43. Bell's Palsy — 100

IX. Neuro-Oncology — 103
- 44. Brain Tumors — 104
- 45. Pituitary Tumors — 106

X. Pain — 109
- 46. Headache — 110
- 47. Migraine — 112
- 48. Tension and Cluster Headache — 114
- 49. Neuropathic Pain — 116

XI. Neuro-Immunology — 119
- 50. Multiple Sclerosis — 120

XII. Movement Disorder — 123
- 51. Parkinson's Disease — 124
- 52. Parkinson Plus Syndromes — 126
- 53. Essential Tremor — 128

XIII. Neurodegenerative Disease — 131
- 54. Dementia — 132

XIV. Sleep Disorders — 137
- 55. Narcolepsy — 138
- 56. Obstructive Sleep Apnea — 140

XV. Pediatric Neurology — 143
- 57. Floppy Baby Syndrome — 144
- 58. Mitochondrial Disorders — 146
- 59. Neurocutaneous Syndromes — 148
- 60. Cerebral Palsy — 150

Appendix — 152

Index — 158

To the Reader

Like most medical students, I started my ward experience head-down and running, eager to finally make contact with real patients. What I found was a confusing world, completely different from anything I had known during the first two years of medical school. New language, foreign abbreviations, and residents too busy to set my bearings straight: Where would I begin?

Pocket textbooks, offering medical knowledge in a convenient and portable package, seemed to be the logical solution. Unfortunately, I found myself spending valuable time sifting through large amounts of text, often not finding the answer to my question, and in the process, missing out on teaching points during rounds!

I designed the SOAP series to provide medical students and house staff with pocket manuals that truly serve their intended purpose: quick accessibility to the most practical clinical information in a user-friendly format. At the inception of this project, I envisioned all of the benefits the SOAP format would bring to the reader:

- Learning through this model reinforces a thought process that is already familiar to students and residents, facilitating easier long-term retention.

- SOAP promotes good communication between physicians and facilitates the teaching/learning process.

- SOAP puts the emphasis back on the patient's clinical problem and not the diagnosis.

- In the age of managed care, SOAP meets the challenge of providing efficiency while maintaining quality.

- As sound medical-legal practice gains attention in physician training, SOAP emphasizes adherence to a documentation style that leaves little room for potential misinterpretation.

Rather than attempting to summarize the contents of a thousand-page textbook into a miniature form, the SOAP series focuses exclusively on guidance through patient encounters. In a typical use, "finding out where to start" or "refreshing your memory" with SOAP books should be possible in less than a minute. Subjects are always confined to two pages and the most important points have been highlighted. Topics have been limited to those problems you will most commonly encounter repeatedly during your training, and contents are grouped according to the hospital or clinic setting. Facts and figures that are not particularly helpful to surviving life on the wards, such as demographics, pathophysiology, and busy tables and graphs, have purposely been omitted (such details are much better studied in a quiet environment using large and comprehensive texts).

Congratulations on your achievements thus far, and I wish you a highly successful medical career!

Peter S. Uzelac, MD, FACOG

Reviewers

Simin Bahrami
4th year student
David Geffen School of Medicine at UCLA
Los Angeles, California

Jessica M. Flynn
3rd year student
Johns Hopkins University School of Medicine
Baltimore, Maryland

Sandy Green
4th year student
Temple University School of Medicine
Philadelphia, Pennsylvania

Susan Merel
4th year student
University of Chicago Pritzker School of Medicine
Chicago, Illinois

Parham Yashar
4th year student
Northwestern University Feinberg School of Medicine
Chicago, Illinois

Randy Young
4th year student
University of California, Davis School of Medicine
Davis, California

Abbreviations

ABG	arterial blood gas
ACA	anterior cerebral artery
ACh	acetylcholine
AD	Alzheimer disease
AED	anti-epileptic drug
AHI	apnea-hypopnea index
AIDS	acquired immunodeficiency syndrome
ALS	amyotrophic lateral sclerosis
AMS	altered mental status
APD	afferent pupillary defect
ASA	acetylsalicylic acid (aspirin)
ATP	adenosine triphosphate
AVM	arteriovenous malformation
AZT	azathioprine
BID	two times daily
BiPAP	bilevel positive airway pressure
BOE	benign occipital epilepsy
BP	blood pressure
BPPV	benign paroxysmal positional vertigo
BRE	benign rolandic epilepsy
BUN	blood urea nitrogen
CBC	complete blood count
CBGD	corticobasal ganglionic degeneration
CC	chief complaint
CDC	Centers for Disease Control
CHF	congestive heart failure
CIDP	chronic inflammatory demyelinating polyradioneuropathy
CJD	Creutzfeldt-Jakob disease
CK	creatine kinase
CMAP	compound muscle action potential
CNS	central nervous system
CP	cerebral palsy
CPAP	continuous positive airway pressure
CPP	cerebral perfusion pressure
CSF	cerebrospinal fluid
CT	computed tomography
CTS	carpal tunnel syndrome
CVP	central venous pressure
CXR	chest x-ray
DDx	differential diagnosis
DM	diabetes mellitus, dermatomyositis
DNR	do not resuscitate
DWI	diffusion weighted image
ECG	electrocardiograph
ED	emergency department
EDS	excessive daytime sleepiness
EEG	electroencephalograph
EITB	enzyme-linked immunotransfer blot

ELISA	enzyme-linked immunosorbent assay
EMG	electromyogram
EOM	extraocular muscle
EP	evoked potential
ESR	erythrocyte sedimentation rate
EtOH	alcohol
FDA	Food and Drug Administration
FHx	family history
FTD	frontotemporal dementia
GBS	Guillain-Barré syndrome
GCS	Glasgow coma scale
GI	gastrointestinal
GTC	generalized tonic-clonic
Hct	hematocrit
HIV	human immunodeficiency virus
HPI	history of present illness
hr(s)	hours
HSV	herpes simplex virus
HTN	hypertension
HV	hyperventilation
IBM	inclusion body myositis
ICA	internal carotid artery
ICH	intracerebral hemorrhage
ICP	intracranial pressure
ICU	intensive care unit
IM	intramuscular
IQ	intelligence quotient
IS	infantile spasms
IV	intravenous
IVIG	intravenous immune globulin
JME	juvenile myoclonic epilepsy
LES	Lambert-Eaton syndrome
LFCN	lateral femoral cutaneous nerve
LGS	Lennox Gastaut syndrome
LOC	loss of consciousness
LP	lumbar puncture
MAO	monoamine oxidase
MAP	mean arterial pressure
MCA	middle cerebral artery
MD	muscular dystrophy
meds	medications
MG	myasthenia gravis
min	minute
MLF	medial longitudinal fasciculus
MRA	magnetic resonance angiography
MRI	magnetic resonance imaging
MRV	magnetic resonance venography
MS	multiple sclerosis
MSA	multiple system atrophy
NCS	nerve conduction studies
NG	nasogastric

NMJ	neuromuscular junction
NPH	normal pressure hydrocephalus
NPO	nothing by mouth
NSAIDs	nonsteroidal anti-inflammatory drugs
OCP	oral contraceptive pill
OSA	obstructive sleep apnea
PaCO$_2$	partial pressure of carbon dioxide in arterial blood
PCA	posterior cerebral artery
PCR	polymerase chain reaction
PD	Parkinson disease
PEO	progressive external ophthalmoplegia
PLMD	periodic limb movement disorder
PM	polymyositis
PMH	past medical history
PML	progressive multifocal encephalitis
PO	by mouth
PPD	purified protein derivative
PPRF	paramedian pontine reticular formation
PRN	as needed
PSG	polysomnography
PSH	past surgical history
PSP	progressive supranuclear palsy
PT	prothrombin time
pt(s)	patient(s)
PTA	prior to admission
PTT	partial thromboplastin time
Q	every
QAC	before every meal
QD	once daily
QHS	every night
QID	four times daily
QOD	every other day
RBC	red blood cells
REM	rapid eye movement
RLS	restless leg syndrome
ROC	reason of consultation
ROS	review of systems
RPR	rapid plasma reagent
SAH	subarachnoid hemorrhage
SC	subcutaneous
SE	status epilepticus
SHx	social history
SSPE	subacute sclerosing panencephalitis
SSRI	selective serotonin reuptake inhibitors
STAT	immediately
SW	Sturge-Weber disease
TB	tuberculosis
TBI	traumatic brain injury
TCD	transcranial Doppler
TIA	transient ischemic attack
TID	three times daily

TLE	temporal lobe epilepsy	
tPA	tissue plasminogen activator	
TS	Tay-Sachs disease	
TSH	thyroid stimulating hormone	
UV	ultraviolet	
VDRL	Venereal Disease Research Laboratory	
VNS	vagal nerve stimulator	
VP	ventriculoperitoneal	
WBC	white blood cell	
wk(s)	week(s)	
y/o	years old	
yr(s)	year(s)	

Normal Lab Values

Blood, Plasma, Serum

Aminotransferase, alanine (ALT, SGPT)	0–35 U/L
Aminotransferase, aspartate (AST, SGOT)	0–35 U/L
Ammonia, plasma	40–80 µg/dL
Amylase, serum	0–130 U/L
Antistreptolysin O titer	Less than 150 units
Bicarbonate, serum	23–28 meq/L
Bilirubin, serum	
Total	0.3–1.2 mg/dL
Direct	0–0.3 mg/dL
Blood gases, arterial (room air)	
Po_2	80–100 mm Hg
Pco_2	35–45 mm Hg
pH	7.38–7.44
Calcium, serum	9–10.5 mg/dL
Carbon dioxide content, serum	23–28 meq/L
Chloride, serum	98–106 meq/L
Cholesterol, total, plasma	150–199 mg/dL (desirable)
Cholesterol, low-density lipoprotein (LDL), plasma	≤130 mg/dL (desirable)
Cholesterol, high-density lipoprotein (HDL), plasma	≥40 mg/dL (desirable)
Complement, serum	
C3	55–120 mg/dL
Total	37–55 U/mL
Copper, serum	70–155 µg/dL
Creatine kinase, serum	30–170 U/L
Creatinine, serum	0.7–1.3 mg/dL
Ethanol, blood	<50 mg/dL
Fibrinogen, plasma	150–350 mg/dL
Folate, red cell	160–855 ng/mL
Folate, serum	2.5–20 ng/mL
Glucose, plasma	
Fasting	70–105 mg/dL
2 hours postprandial	<140 mg/dL
Iron, serum	60–160 µg/dL
Iron binding capacity, serum	250–460 µg/dL
Lactate dehydrogenase, serum	60–100 U/L
Lactic acid, venous blood	6–16 mg/dL
Lead, blood	<40 µg/dL
Lipase, serum	<95 U/L

Magnesium, serum	1.5–2.4 mg/dL
Manganese, serum	0.3–0.9 ng/mL
Methylmalonic acid, serum	150–370 nmol/L
Osmolality plasma	275–295 mOsm/kg H_2O
Phosphatase, acid, serum	0.5–5.5 U/L
Phosphatase, alkaline, serum	36–92 U/L
Phosphorus, inorganic, serum	3–4.5 mg/dL
Potassium, serum	3.5–5 meq/L
Protein, serum	
Total	6.0–7.8 g/dL
Albumin	3.5–5.5 g/dL
Globulins	2.5–3.5 g/dL
Alpha$_1$	0.2–0.4 g/dL
Alpha$_2$	0.5–0.9 g/dL
Beta	0.6–1.1 g/dL
Gamma	0.7–1.7 g/dL
Rheumatoid factor	<40 U/mL
Sodium, serum	136–145 meq/L
Triglycerides	<250 mg/dL (desirable)
Urea nitrogen, serum	8–20 mg/dL
Uric acid, serum	2.5–8 mg/dL
Vitamin B_{12}, serum	200–800 pg/mL

Cerebrospinal Fluid

Cell count	0–5 cells/μL
Glucose (less than 40% of simultaneous plasma concentration is abnormal)	40–80 mg/dL
Protein	15–60 mg/dL
Pressure (opening)	70–200 cm H_2O

Endocrine

Adrenocorticotropin (ACTH)	9–52 pg/mL
Aldosterone, serum	
Supine	2–5 ng/dL
Standing	7–20 ng/dL
Aldosterone, urine	5–19 μg/24 h
Cortisol	
Serum 8 AM	8–20 μg/dL
5 PM	3–13 μg/dL
1 h after cosyntropin usually ≥ 8 μg/dL above baseline	>18 μg/dL
overnight suppression test	<5 μg/dL
Urine free cortisol	<90 μg/24 h

Estradiol, serum	
Male	10–30 pg/mL
Female	
Cycle day 1–10	50–100 pmol/L
Cycle day 11–20	50–200 pmol/L
Cycle day 21–30	70–150 pmol/L
Estriol, urine	>12 mg/24 h
Follicle-stimulating hormone, serum	
Male (adult)	5–15 mU/mL
Female	
Follicular or luteal phase	5–20 mU/mL
Midcycle peak	30–50 mU/mL
Postmenopausal	>35 mU/mL
Insulin, serum (fasting)	5–20 mU/L
17-ketosteroids, urine	
Male	8–22 mg/24 h
Female	Up to 15 μg/24 h
Luteinizing hormone, serum	
Male	3–15 mU/mL (3–15 U/L)
Female	
Follicular or luteal phase	5–22 mU/mL
Midcycle peak	30–250 mU/mL
Postmenopausal	>30 mU/mL
Parathyroid hormone, serum	10–65 pg/mL
Progesterone	
Luteal	3–30 ng/mL
Follicular	<1 ng/mL
Prolactin, serum	
Male	<15 ng/mL
Female	<20 ng/mL
Testosterone, serum	
Adult male	300–1200 ng/dL
Female	20–75 ng/dL
Thyroid function tests (normal ranges vary)	
Thyroid iodine (^{131}I) uptake	10% to 30% of administered dose at 24 h
Thyroid-stimulating hormone (TSH)	0.5–5.0 μU/mL
Thyroxine (T4), serum	
Total	5–12 pg/dL
Free	0.9–2.4 ng/dL
Free T4 index	4–11

Triiodothyronine, resin (T3)	25%–35%
Triiodothyronine, serum (T3)	70–195 ng/dL
Vitamin D	
1,25-dihydroxy, serum	25–65 pg/mL
25-hydroxy, serum	15–80 ng/mL

Gastrointestinal

Fecal urobilinogen	40–280 mg/24 h
Gastrin, serum	0–180 pg/mL
Lactose tolerance test	
Increase in plasma glucose	>15 mg/dL
Lipase, ascitic fluid	<200 U/L
Secretin-cholecystokinin pancreatic function	>80 meq/L of HCO_3 in at least 1 specimen collected over 1 h
Stool fat	<5 g/d on a 100-g fat diet
Stool nitrogen	<2 g/d
Stool weight	<200 g/d

Hematology

Activated partial thromboplastin time	25–35 s
Bleeding time	<10 min
Coagulation factors, plasma	
Factor I	150–350 mg/dL
Factor II	60%–150% of normal
Factor V	60%–150% of normal
Factor VII	60%–150% of normal
Factor VIII	60%–150% of normal
Factor IX	60%–150% of normal
Factor X	60%–150% of normal
Factor XI	60%–150% of normal
Factor XII	60%–150% of normal
Erythrocyte count	4.2–5.9 million cells/μL
Erythropoietin	<30 mU/mL
D-dimer	<0.5 μg/mL
Ferritin, serum	15–200 ng/mL
Glucose-6-phosphate dehydrogenase, blood	5–15 U/g Hgb
Haptoglobin, serum	50–150 mg/dL
Hematocrit	
Male	41%–51%
Female	36%–47%
Hemoglobin, blood	
Male	14–17 g/dL
Female	12–16 g/dL

Hemoglobin, plasma	0.5–5 mg/dL
Leukocyte alkaline phosphatase	15–40 mg of phosphorus liberated/h per 10^{10} cells
Score	13–130/100 polymorphonuclear neutrophils and band forms
Leukocyte count	
Nonblacks	4000–10,000/μL
Blacks	3500–10,000/μL
Lymphocytes	
CD4+ cell count	640–1175/μL
CD8+ cell count	335–875/μL
CD4:CD8 ratio	1.0–4.0
Mean corpuscular hemoglobin (MCH)	28–32 pg
Mean corpuscular hemoglobin concentration (MCHC)	32–36 g/dL
Mean corpuscular volume (MCV)	80–100 fL
Platelet count	150,000–350,000/μL
Protein C activity, plasma	67%–I 31%
Protein C resistance	2.2–2.6
Protein S activity, plasma	82%–144%
Prothrombin time	11–13 s
Reticulocyte count	0.5%–1.5% of erythrocytes
Absolute	23,000–90,000 cells/μL
Schilling test (oral administration of radioactive cobalamin-labeled vitamin B_{12})	8.5%–28% excreted in urine per 24–48 h
Sedimentation rate, erythrocyte (Westergren)	
Male	0–15 mm/h
Female	0–20 mm/h
Volume, blood	
Plasma	
Male	25–44 mL/kg body weight
Female	28–43 mL/kg body weight
Erythrocyte	
Male	25–35 mL/kg body weight
Female	20–30 mL/kg body weight

Urine

Amino acids	200–400 mg/24 h
Amylase	6.5–48.1 U/h
Calcium	100–300 mg/d on unrestricted diet
Chloride	80–250 meq/d (varies with intake)

Copper	0–100 µg/24 h
Creatine	
Male	4–40 mg/24 h
Female	0–100 mg/24 h
Creatinine	15–25 mg/kg per 24 h
Creatinine clearance	90–140 mL/min
Osmolality	38–1400 mOsm/kg H_2O
Phosphate, tubular resorption	79%–94% (0.79–0.94) of filtered load
Potassium	25–100 meq/24 h (varies with intake)
Protein	<100 mg/24 h
Sodium	100–260 meq/24h (varies with intake)
Uric acid	250–750 mg/24 h (varies with diet)
Urobilinogen	0.05–2.5 mg/24 h

I
Evaluation

S **Neurologic history**

Focus on the pt's chief complaint (CC) or the reason of consultation (ROC). The complete history consists of CC/ROC, history of present illness (HPI), past medical history (PMH), past surgical history (PSH), family history (FHx), social history (SHx), allergies (ALL), medications (meds), and review of systems (ROS). This is the order history should be presented.

The HPI is the most important part of history and should contain all the information relevant to the CC/ROC, including information from other parts of history (e.g., In a pt presenting with stroke symptoms, PMH of hypertension/diabetes mellitus, and SHx of smoking should be included under HPI).

The history is best presented in chronological fashion, starting at earliest time pertaining to the CC/ROC. For example, a typical Guillain-Barré syndrome pt history would be, "This is a 30-year-old white male in an usual state of health until 3 wks prior to admission (PTA) when he developed upper respiratory infection symptoms that lasted 5 days. About 3 days PTA pt began having weakness involving both lower extremities, progressing to both upper extremities."

O **Neurologic exam**

For beginners, a complete neurologic exam should be performed on all pts in a systematic manner to avoid missing critical findings. As one gains more experience, exams can be focused and tailored to the clinical setting.

The following is a list of basic components of neurologic exam. Under each chapter additional focus and special tests will be mentioned.

Mental status and higher cortical functions
Level of consciousness: alert, drowsy, stuporous, obtunded, comatose
Orientation: to person, place, time
Concentration: serial 7, spell "WORLD" and "DLROW"
Memory: ask recent major news, name president, three objects 5-min recall
Speech: fluency, repetition, naming, comprehension, reading, writing
Visual-spatial: draw clock, copy figures
Mini Mental Status Examination is a quick and easy way to assess and score mental status.

Cranial nerves
Olfactory: smell
Optic: optic disks, pupillary response (afferent), visual acuity, visual fields
Oculomotor: pupillary responses (efferent), levator palpebrae, eye adduction, up and down gaze
Trochlear: eye down gaze and intorsion
Trigeminal: facial sensory, corneal reflex (afferent)
Abducent: eye abduction
Facial: facial muscles, eye closure, corneal reflex (efferent), chorda tympani (taste of anterior one third of tongue), hyperacusis (stapedius)
Vestibular: hearing, balance, oculocephalic reflex (afferent)
Glossopharyngeal/vagus: gag reflex, palate elevation
Spinal accessory: shoulder shrug, turn head against resistance
Hypoglossal: tongue protrusion

Motor exam
Observe for any involuntary movements
Tone: passive range of motion of elbow, wrist, knees, and shoulders
Bulk: evidence of hypertrophy or atrophy
Power: 0 (no contraction), 1 (contraction but no movement), 2 (horizontal movements but cannot overcome gravity), 3 (able to overcome gravity), 4 (not able to overcome resistance), 5 (normal)

Reflexes: 0 (absent), 1 (decreased), 2 (normal), 3 (brisk), 4 (with clonus). Check biceps, triceps, brachioradialis, knee, and ankle. Babinski reflex.

Sensory exam
Light touch, pin prick, temperature: use disposable pins and cold surfaces of tuning fork
Vibration: use 128-Hz tuning fork, compare distal to proximal
Proprioception: ask pt whether fingers/toes moved up and down, Romberg
Two-point discrimination: on hand
Cortical sensory function: graphesthesia, stereognosis, double simultaneous stimulation

Coordination and Gait
- Finger-to-nose test and heel-to-shin
- Standing
- Tandem walk
- Rapid alternating movement
- Walking

A **Neurologic assessment**

After history and physical, the physician should first come up with *anatomic localization* of the disease process.

The anatomic sites in neurology, starting from the most periphery, include:
- Muscle (type 1, type 2)
- Neuromuscular junction (presynaptic, synaptic, postsynaptic)
- Peripheral nerves (sensory—large vs. small fiber, motor, autonomic mixed)
- Plexus (trunk, division, cord)
- Nerve roots (C1–S5)
- Spinal cord (anterior, posterior, central, hemi, transverse)
- Brainstem/cerebellum (lateral/medial/anterior/posterior medullary, pons, midbrain)
- Subcortical structures (subarachnoid space, thalamus, basal ganglia, internal capsule, corona radiata, white matters)
- Cerebral cortex (gray matters of frontal, temporal, parietal, occipital)

From the exam it is often not possible to pinpoint where the disease process is, but attempts should be made to localize the lesion to the most general areas (e.g., central vs. peripheral, muscle vs. nerve, cortical vs. subcortical).

After anatomic localization, one can generate the *differential diagnosis* or etiology involving that particular area. A good mnemonic to remember is **VITAMINS:**

- Vascular: infarct, hemorrhage, malformations, hypoperfusion, hypoxic
- Infectious: viral, bacterial, fungal, parasitic, prion
- Traumatic: subdural hematoma, EPH, contusion, fracture, intracerebral hemorrhage, diffuse axonal injury
- Autoimmune: multiple sclerosis, systemic lupus erythematosus, sarcoid, post-infectious
- Metabolic: thyroid, hepatic, uremic, electrolytes, endocrine
- Iatrogenic: drugs, toxins, heavy metals, organophosphate
- Neoplastic: tumors, paraneoplastic syndromes
- Seizures

P **Determine the best treatment and supportive care for the pt**
Decide based on knowledge of the disease, its natural course, and prognosis, as well as pt's needs, goals, and expectations.

II
Strokes and Critical Care

When did the stroke happen?

If the symptoms started within 3 hrs, pt is a candidate for thrombolytic therapy. The diagnosis needs to be established ASAP.

Does the pt have risk factors for stroke?
Hypertension (HTN), diabetes mellitus (DM), heart disease, hyperlipidemia, smoking, family history of cerebrovascular accident, male, age > 65, black, carotid artery disease, history of transient ischemic attacks/stroke, high RBC count.

Perform a general physical exam
Assess airways, breathing, and circulation.
Auscultate heart for murmurs and arrhythmia. Check carotids for bruits.

Determine the mental status
Pt remains awake and alert in small vessel or lacunar stroke
Confusion suggests large vessel strokes in frontal, temporal, or parietal lobes
Stupor and coma usually indicate stroke involving the reticular activating system in brainstem, or both hemispheres with mass effect midline shift and herniation.

Does the pt have any signs of cortical stroke (the 4 As)?
Aphasia: assess comprehension, naming, repetition
Apraxia: pretend to brush teeth, light a match, use scissors
Agnosia: ask pt to identify a small object in hand with eyes closed
Anopsia: check visual field cuts

Does the pt have any signs of brainstem and cerebellar stroke (the 4 Ds) (posterior circulation)?
Diplopia: check for extraocular movements
Dysarthria: assess the smoothness of pt's speech
Dysphagia: check for gag, ask for any swallowing difficulty
Dysmetria: do finger-nose-finger testing, rapid alternating movement

What is the pattern of weakness and numbness?
Large vessels stroke involves the motor and sensory homunculus, which are spread over a large surface area. Therefore the degree of weakness will be different among face, arm, and leg (e.g., middle cerebral artery [MCA] stroke will affect face and arm more than leg and anterior cerebral artery [ACA] stroke will affect leg much more than arm and face).
Small vessel strokes in internal capsule, thalamus, and pontine stroke affects the descending motor/sensory fibers that are densely packed. They will tend to produce same degree of weakness/numbness in face, arm, and leg.

Obtain head imaging
Head imaging needs to be done on all acute stroke pts. The only way to tell whether a stroke is ischemic or hemorrhagic is by imaging.
Head CT is very sensitive in diagnosing hemorrhagic stroke but not ischemic stroke. CT can remain negative up to 24 hrs after an ischemic stroke.
CT is not sensitive for brainstem/cerebellum strokes due to bony artifacts in the posterior fossa.
MRI is very sensitive in detecting strokes; however, it does not distinguish hemorrhage versus infarct as well as CT, and it is not available in every hospital.

Ischemic stroke
Stroke is the third most common cause of death in U.S. Incidence is approximately 750,000/yr.
"Stroke" refers to brain injury caused by vascular mechanism. The two major categories are ischemic and hemorrhagic. For ischemic, the three major causes, in order of frequency, are:

- Thrombosis: blood clot superimposed on an atherosclerotic plaque
- Embolism: when a clot, plaque, or agglutinated platelets from the heart or proximal arteries occlude an intracranial artery.
- Systemic reduction in flow: seen in cardiac arrest or shock, lead to border zone infarcts.

When evaluating stroke, categorize stroke into (1) cortical vs. subcortical and (2) anterior vs. posterior circulation.

1. Cortical and subcortical stroke can be differentiated by the presence of 4 As (see above). In general, cortical strokes are *large vessel strokes* and subcortical strokes are *small vessel strokes* (a.k.a. *lacunar infarct*). Large vessel strokes involve the major branches of MCA, ACA, and posterior cerebral artery (PCA). Small vessel strokes affect the deep penetrating vessels in the basal ganglia, thalamus, internal capsule, and brainstem.
2. Anterior (MCA, ACA) and posterior (vertebral basilar, PCA) circulation stroke can be differentiated by the 4 Ds.

Cortical and posterior circulation stokes have higher morbidity and mortality. They require longer hospital stays and higher level of care.

P **Consider thrombolytics therapy**
If stroke is < 3 hrs and there is no contraindication, then tissue plasminogen activator (tPA) is indicated (see below).
Infuse total of 0.9 mg/kg, 10% as bolus over 1 min and the remainder over 60 min. Monitor BP Q 15 min the first 2 hrs, Q 30 min the next 6 hrs, and Q 60 min the next 18 hrs. Keep BP below 185/100 mm Hg.
tPA contraindications include minor or improving stroke symptoms, seizure at onset of stroke, other stroke within previous 3 months, major surgery in previous 14 days, known history of intracerebral hemorrhage, systolic BP > 185 mm Hg, diastolic BP > 110 mm Hg, GI or urinary tract bleed within 21 days, elevated PT and PTT, platelet < 100,000, glucose < 50 or > 400.

Start stroke prophylaxis medication
For thrombotic strokes, start antiplatelet meds (ASA, Plavix, or Aggrenox).
For embolic strokes, consider anticoagulation with heparin and coumadin.

Monitor blood pressure in first 48–72 hrs after stroke
Cerebral perfusion pressure = mean arterial pressure (MAP) − intracerebral pressure. MAP needs to be maintained to perfuse the brain.
Most pts presenting with acute stroke will have high blood pressure. It is a normal physiologic response to decreased brain perfusion. There is no need to treat it unless it is very high (i.e., MAP > 130). Use IV meds such as labetalol and hydralazine to bring down BP. Do not use PO BP meds. Avoid nitrates because they can cause vasodilation in brain and increase intracranial pressure.

Initiate stroke workup
Look for correctable causes such as thyroid disease, syphilis, and hypercoagulable state.
For pts < 55 without known risk factors, perform a young stroke workup. (See p. 14.)
In case of large vessel stroke, echocardiogram with bubble study should be performed. The bubble study is to look for patent foramen ovale.
Carotid ultrasound should be performed in all stroke pts, especially pts with large vessel stroke. Carotid endarterectomy is recommended for stenosis > 70%.

Risk factor modification
Modifiable risk factors include HTN, DM, hyperlipidemia, and smoking. Treat these risk factors aggressively.
Long-term goal: BP < 135/85 mm Hg; HgbA1c < 6; low-density lipoprotein < 100; smoking cessation

8 Hemorrhagic Stroke — Strokes and Critical Care

Does the pt have risk factors of hemorrhagic stroke?
By far the most common cause of intracerebral hemorrhage is chronic hypertension. Other risk factors include diabetes, vascular malformations, bleeding diatheses, and drug abuse.

Are there symptoms of increased intracranial pressure?
Hemorrhagic strokes are more likely to cause increased intracranial pressure (ICP) due to mass effect from the hematoma. Symptoms of increased ICP include headache, nausea/vomiting, and lethargy.

Assess ABCs (airway, breathing, and circulation) and vital signs
Pt may be comatose. Establish airway.
Hypopnea and apnea can occur if brainstem is being compressed.
Blood pressure is usually elevated > 180/100 mm Hg.

Look for signs of elevated ICP
Papilledema, subhyaloid retinal hemorrhage, unilateral or bilateral CN6 palsy, restricted upward gaze (sun setting eyes). See chapter on ICP.

Perform neurologic exam
Perform a neurologic exam to find out if it is a stroke and where the lesion is located.

Send routine labs
Chemistry, CBC, urinalysis, toxicology screen, PT, and PTT

Obtain head CT scan without contrast
Quickest and most sensitive test to diagnose intracerebral hemorrhage (ICH)
Also check for radiologic evidence of intraventricular blood, mass effect, and midline shift.

A

Intracerebral hemorrhage
ICH accounts for 10% to 15% of all strokes.
It has a higher mortality rate than ischemic stroke.
The most common cause of ICH is chronic hypertension. The vessels affected are the small vessels. Microaneurysms form at weak points as the vessels degenerate. ICH occurs when one of the microaneurysms ruptures. The hematoma exerts pressure on adjacent microaneurysms causing them to rupture as well. Bleeding stops when tissue turgor matches the intravascular blood pressure.

The most common sites of ICH, in order of decreasing frequency, are basal ganglia, deep white matter, thalamus, pons, and cerebellum.

Another common cause of ICH is cerebral amyloid angiopathy, a degenerative vascular disease seen in elderly. β-Amyloid deposits in the arteries in the gray matter of the brain, making the area more prone to bleed.
Other causes of ICH to consider include:
- Cocaine and amphetamine
- Bleeding diatheses such as thrombocytopenia, hemophilia, and hypoprothrombinemia from cirrhosis or anticoagulation therapy.
- Vascular malformations such as arteriovenous malformations, aneurysm, and cavernous hemangioma. Look for history of headaches and seizures.

Admit to ICU
Most pts with ICH are in critical condition. Most are obtunded and require intubation for airway protection.
Put pt on bed rest. Sedate pt if needed.
NPO except meds because risk of aspiration is high.

Manage ICP
One of the keys to achieve minimal brain damage from ICH is carefully control ICP. Refer to the chapter on ICP management.

Correct coagulopathies, if any
Give fresh-frozen plasma and vitamin K for prolonged PT and PTT.
Give platelet transfusion of thrombocytopenia (platelets < 50).

Blood pressure management
BP is usually out of control. It is not unusual to see systolic BP > 220 and diastolic BP greater than 140 mm Hg.
Goal of BP control should be mean arterial pressure (MAP) less than 110. Avoid rapid decrease in BP.
Common PRN anti-hypertensive medication used in ICH include:
- Labetalol: give 5–10 mg IV Q 10 min PRN MAP > 110
- Hydralazine: 10 mg IV Q 1 to 2 hrs PRN MAP > 110
- Enalapril 1.25 mg IV Q 6 hrs PRN MAP > 110

Sometimes BP is volatile and it is best to use a drip to maintain steady BP.
- Nicardipine IV start 5 mg/hr and titrate by 2.5 mg/hr Q 5 to 15 min to maintain MAP < 110. Maximum rate is 15 mg/hr.

Consult neurosurgery
Unlike traumatic brain hemorrhage, hemorrhagic stroke does not respond well to surgical hematoma evacuation.
However if pt has a large hematoma with mass effect and impending herniation, surgical intervention is indicated.
In case of bleeding into the ventricles, ventriculostomy drain should be inserted to prevent hydrocephalus and at the same time monitor intracranial pressure.
In case of bleeding in the posterior fossa (brainstem and cerebellum), craniotomy is usually required because the risk of brainstem compression and cessation of vital cardiac and respiratory functions.

Initiate physical, occupational, and speech/swallow therapy when stable
Pt surviving ICH usually recovers better than ischemic stroke. Arrange inpatient rehabilitation if possible. Most pts will be stable enough to undergo physical therapy 5 to 7 days post bleed.
Do swallow evaluation before start pt on PO diet. If pt fails, start tube feeding through nasogastric (NG) tube.

Discuss plan with family
Often pt will have severe residual neurologic deficit. It is the neurologist's job to give an expected functional capacity and explain to the family member.
Discuss DNR (do not resuscitate) status.
If long-term care is required, have family or social worker initiate placement finding early.
If pt cannot protect his/her airway, will need to convert endotracheal tube to tracheotomy.
If pt is unable to swallow, will need to convert NG to percutaneous endoscopic gastrostomy tube.
If pt is likely to remain in permanent vegetative state, discuss withdrawal of care with family.

S **Does the pt have these common symptoms of transient ischemic attacks (TIA)?**
- Weakness and/or numbness in face, arm, and/or leg
- Dizziness
- Transient monocular blindness (amaurosis fugax)
- Imbalance
- Confusion
- Slurred speech
- Double vision
- Hemianopia
- Aphasia

Does the pt have any risk factors for stroke?
Hypertension (HTN), diabetes mellitus (DM), hyperlipidemia, smoking, and family history.

How long did the symptom last?
By definition TIA lasts < 24 hrs, longer than that it is a stroke
However more than 90% of TIAs last less than 10 min
If the symptom lasts > 24 hrs and then resolves within 3 wks, it is called *residual ischemic neurologic deficit*. The risk of subsequent stroke is increased to six times that of the normal population.

How many episodes and how often did the pt experience?
If pt experiences the same symptoms multiple times, it usually indicates critical narrowing of the lumen of the involved artery by an atherosclerotic plaque with superimposing thrombus.

What is the pattern of symptoms?
If pt experiences different symptoms corresponding to different vascular territories (e.g., hemianopia and hemiparesis), then it may indicate an embolic source distal to the take-off of both arteries.

Perform a general physical and neurologic exam
Assess vital signs
Check for carotid bruits
Listen for heart murmurs
For pt with amaurosis fugax, funduscopic exam may reveal embolus in one of the retinal arteries.
Assess for any neurologic deficits. If the pt has persistent deficit, then the diagnosis is stroke, not TIA.

Obtain lab tests
Routine labs chemistry panel, CBC, urinalysis, PT, PTT.
Toxicology screen. Cocaine has high association with stroke/TIA.
Elevation of ESR may suggest endocarditis or temporal arteritis.
ECG to look for atrial fibrillation and evidence of myocardial infarction.

Obtain head imaging
Head CT is usually obtained in the emergency department and is negative in TIA.
Brain MRI with DWI is very sensitive in picking up small strokes. If brain MRI shows acute infarct then pt has a stroke, not TIA.

Transient Ischemic Attack
TIA is very common. Annual incidence is estimated at 500,000. The actual number maybe higher because many pts with TIA do not come to medical attention.
It is defined as a neurologic deficit lasting less than 24 hrs that is attributed to focal cerebral or retinal ischemia.
It is a clinical diagnosis. Laboratory and radiologic studies are often non-revealing. Good history is the key to diagnose TIA.
TIA is often viewed as precursor to stroke. The 90-day risk of stroke is approximately 20%. Half of those strokes occurred in the first 2 days after TIA.
Therefore it is imperative to recognize and diagnose TIA early and initiated stroke prevention therapy.

Admit pt to hospital
As mentioned previously, the chance of having a stroke is the highest in the first 2 days. It is best to admit a TIA pt to the hospital, observe, complete the workup, and initiate treatment.

Determine the location of stenosis or embolic source
Use clinical judgment to determine whether it is a thrombotic vs. embolic event and location of the lesion.
Transthoracic echocardiogram should be performed on all TIA pts.
If pt does not have A-fib, but a cardiac embolic source is strongly suspected, then transesophageal echocardiogram should be performed.
Ultrasound of carotid arteries should be performed on all pts. The most common site for carotid artery stenosis is at the bifurcation of common carotid artery.
If vertebral-basilar and posterior cerebral artery TIA are suspected, MRA or CT angiogram should be performed.

Consider carotid endarterectomy
For pts who have had a stroke or TIA and > 70% stenosis in the ipsilateral carotid artery, a study has shown benefit of carotid endarterectomy over medical treatment. The 2-year ipsilateral stroke risk is 9% for surgical vs. 26% for medical treatment.
This does not apply to stenosis less than 50%, for which medical treatment is recommended.

Start stroke prophylaxis
For cardioembolic, start anticoagulation with heparin.
For non-cardioembolic cause, start antiplatelet therapy with ASA, clopidogrel, Aggrenox, or ticlopidine.

Risk-factor management
Control HTN with goal < 135/85 mm Hg
Control DM with goal of HgbA1c < 6
Control lipids with total cholesterol < 200 and low density lipoprotein < 100
Smoking cessation
Diet and exercise
Stress management

Cerebral Venous Thrombosis

S **Are there any risk factors for venous thrombosis?**
Common risk factors for venous thrombosis include:
- Pregnancy, postpartum period, and history of unexplained abortions
- Drugs such as oral contraceptive, corticosteroids, heparin (heparin-induced thrombocytopenia)
  - Hypercoagulable state
  - Dehydration
  - Malignancy
  - Sinus and ear infections
  - Nephrotic syndrome

Does the pt have symptoms of venous thrombosis?
Most common presentation is acute or subacute onset of headache. The headache is often associated with raised intracranial pressure and is often worsened by Valsalva or lying flat.
Other symptoms of ↑ intracranial pressure (ICP) include nausea/vomiting, visual changes such as double vision, blurry vision, and obscuration of vision.
Pts with newly diagnosed pseudotumor cerebri should undergo evaluation to rule out lateral sinus thrombosis.
Pt may or may not have focal neurologic symptom such as hemi-weakness and numbness.
Seizures
Confusion

O **Assess the mental status**
Mental status can range from normal to stupor and coma. Coma results from large vein thrombosis causing herniation and/or compression of brainstem or bilateral cerebral hemisphere.

Check for signs of infection
Often venous thrombosis is triggered by concurrent infections in the head and neck. Look for evidence of scalp abscess, sinusitis, and otitis media.
Check neck stiffness, Brudzinski's, and Kernig's signs for meningitis.

Assess the cranial nerves
Papilledema and CN6 palsies are associated with raised ICP.
Involvement of CN3, CN5, and CN6 is consistent with cavernous sinus thrombosis. Look for dilated pupil, ophthalmoplegia, and diminished corneal reflex and decreased facial sensation (V1 and V2 distribution).
Involvement of CN9, CN10, CN11, and CN12 is suggestive of jugular foramen syndrome when the jugular vein is thrombosed.

Check for other focal neurologic signs
Focal neurologic signs such as hemiparesis, hemisensory loss, and aphasia can occur with the associated cortical vein thrombosis.
Superior sagittal thrombosis can involve one or both medial frontal lobe(s), where the leg homonuculus lies. Unilateral or bilateral lower extremity weakness can be seen.

Obtain labs
Chemistry panel, CBC with differential, urinalysis, liver function tests, PT, PTT
Do urine pregnancy test on females in childbearing age
Anti-nuclear antiboies and ESR to screen for possible systemic lupus erythematosus, vasculitis, and other autoimmune conditions
Hypercoagulable workup if no obvious cause is identified. These tests include proteins C and S, antithrombin III, factor V Leiden, lupus anticoagulant, antiphospholipid, and anticardiolipin antibodies. They are expensive tests; do not order indiscriminately on all pts.

Obtain brain imaging study
Head CT should be done in emergency room situation to rule out hemorrhage and herniation. Look for:
- Empty delta sign—flow void in posterior sagittal sinus from superior sagittal sinus thrombosis.
- Corkscrew sign—the tributary veins resembles "corkscrew" appearance after venous thrombosis is established.

MRI with MRV should be ordered to visualize the extent of brain parenchymal damage and to visualize the venous flow system. It is more sensitive than CT scan but is not 100%.

Digital subtraction angiography is the gold standard in establishing the diagnosis but it is not available in all centers.

Venous thrombosis
Represent about 2% of all strokes.

It can occur at any age from childhood to old age. The three most common groups are:
1. Infants and young children: usually from dehydration, marasmus, meningitis, sinusitis
2. Young premenopausal women: oral contraceptive use, pregnancy, and peripartum (especially during the third trimester)
3. Elderly: result of malignancies and dehydration

The most common sites of venous thrombosis are superior sagittal sinus, lateral sinus, cavernous sinus, and straight sinus.

The blood to the face, ear, and scalp are drained via the emissary veins to the draining sinuses. Scalp infections tend to cause superior sagittal sinus thrombosis. Facial infections cause cavernous sinus thrombosis. Otitis media causes lateral sinus thrombosis.

Stabilize pt first
Intubate if pt not able to protect airway
Address raised ICP and herniation issues. (See Raised ICP p. 20).

Start heparin
Studies have shown benefit of anticoagulation in venous thrombosis. Initiate therapy as soon as possible.

Start with loading dose of 80 unit/kg and then continue at 18 unit/kg/hr. Check PTT Q 6 hrs. PTT goal is two times control.

Start warfarin after PTT is therapeutic. Warfarin is to be continued for 3 to 6 months.

Address the underlying cause of venous thrombosis
Start antibiotics if evidence of infection.
Hydrate with normal saline or lactate ringer if dehydrated.
If pt is hypercoagulable then anticoagulate with warfarin.

Initiate physical therapy/occupational therapy/speech rehabilitation after pt is in stable condition
With modern therapy, mortality from venous thrombosis is approximately 10%.
Pts who survive usually have good neurologic functional recovery.

Stroke in Children and Young Adults

S **What is the age of the pt?**
Stroke is a disease of elderly; however, it is not uncommon to see strokes in children and young adults. Whenever a stroke occurs in a pt younger than 45 years of age, the underlying cause must be carefully sought and adressed.

Are the concurrent chronic illness?
Certain illnesses in young pts predispose them to having stroke:
- Heart disease, such as patent foramen ovale, rheumatic, prosthetic valve
- Sickle cell anemia, polycythemia
- Hereditary metabolic disease, such as mitochondrial disorders, homocystinuria, and Fabry's disease
- Autoimmune diseases, such as lupus, connective tissue disease
- Malignancies

For female pts, is there use of oral contraceptives and pregnancy?
Estrogen alters the coagulability of blood. Women taking oral contraceptive pills (OCP) with high estrogen content have increased risk of stroke, particularly those who are over age 35, those who smoke cigarettes, and those who have hypertension or migraine.
The use of progestin-only OCP has not been associated with an increased risk of stroke.
The risk of stroke increases during pregnancy and postpartum period. Risk is 6.2 per 100,000, but doubles with each advance in age from 25 to 29, 30 to 39, and 40 to 49 years.

Does the pt have any neck pain or trauma to the neck?
Carotid and vertebral artery dissection causes pain in the neck in addition to focal neurologic symptoms.
The most common cause for arterial dissection is trauma to the neck. The trauma can be as minor, such as that in chiropractic manipulation, and can be as severe, as in whiplash.

Was there headache associated with stroke onset?
Migraine is a known cause for stroke, especially in women and in those with an underlying hypercoagulable state.
The risk of stroke increases with the use of triptans.

Get detailed family history
Some hereditary diseases may present as stroke the first symptom.

Ask about use of illicit drugs and sexual history
Cocaine is associated with both ischemic and hemorrhagic strokes.
Neurosyphilis is well known to cause strokes in young adult.

 Perform a general physical and neurologic exam
Please refer to Stroke (p. 6) for basic evaluation of stroke

Labs and studies that should be ordered:
Chemistry panel, CBC, PT, PTT, urinalysis, liver function tests
Both urine and serum toxicology screen
Thyroid-stimulating hormone, RPR, ESR, antinuclear antibody, homocystine
ECG, CXR
2-D ± 3-D echocardiogram with bubble study to look for thrombus and patent foramen ovale
MRI/MRA of brain with contrast
If suspected, cerebral angiogram to look for fibromuscular dysplasia, moyamoya, vasculitis, vascular malformations

Proteins C and S, antithrombin levels should be checked, particularly in venous stroke. Their levels decrease during acute stroke so no need to check until 2 months after. Anti-phospholipid antibody, lupus anticoagulant, anti-cardiolipin antibody, cryoglobulin

Stroke in children and young adults
The most common stroke etiologies by age group are:
1. Newborn: hypoxia in utero or peripartum, congenital brain malformations, matrix hemorrhage, cardiopulmonary failure
2. Infant and children: congenital heart disease and paradoxical embolism, moya-moya, rheumatic fever, systemic lupus erythematosus, endocarditis, sickle cell anemia, mitochondrial disorders, homocystinuria, Fabry's disease
3. Adolescent and young adults: Arterial dissection, moyamoya, antiphospholipid syndrome, factor V Leiden mutation, proteins C and S and antithrombin deficiency, sickle cell anemia, polycythemia, migraine, pregnancy, OCP, cocaine, syphilis, valvular heart disease, vascular malformation, connective tissue diseases, leukemia and lymphoma
4. Middle age adults: Same as young adults plus: atherosclerosis, fibromuscular dysplasia, hypertensive intracerebral hemorrhage (ICH), ruptured aneurysm

Proceed with care for acute stroke
Refer to chapters on stroke and ICH. For young pts, the acute care is the same. The goal is to minimize brain damage.

Start stroke prevention medication
Depending on the etiology found, pt may or may not need stroke prophylaxis with antiplatelet or anticoagulation medications.

If stroke is due to drug use such as OCP or cocaine, remove the offending agent. Be sure to perform hypercoagulability workup because they may have underlying disease only brought out by OCP or cocaine.

If the hypercoagulability workup results are positive, pt will need to undergo anticoagulation therapy.

For arterial dissection, heparin should be started and continue with coumadin for many months until repeat angiogram shows resolution of dissection.

For a hypercoagulable state such as pregnancy, anticoagulation needs to be started and maintained until at least 6 weeks postpartum. Heparin is preferred because it can be turned off quickly during delivery.

If stroke is due to hyperviscosity states such as sickle cell disease or polycythemia, antiplatelet therapy with ASA ± clopidogrel or Persantine should be adequate. Pt will need to have optimal control of underlying disease.

Initiate inpatient physical therapy program
Young stroke pts have a remarkable ability to recover from neurologic injuries. The unaffected hemisphere often picks up the functions normally carried out by the damaged contralateral areas. This is especially true for children. A multidisciplinary rehabilitation program involving physical, occupation, and speech therapy will make the biggest difference in these pt's lives.

Subarachnoid Hemorrhage

S **Does the pt have the symptoms of subarachnoid hemorrhage (SAH)?**
Classis symptom is sudden onset of "worse headache of my life"
Nausea and vomiting
Photophobia and visual changes
Neck and back pain
Seizures
Sometimes followed by loss of consciousness

What was the pt doing when the headache started?
SAH usually occurs while pt is active and exerting rather than during sleep (e.g., sexual intercourse, straining at stool, and lifting heavy objects).

Does the pt have any risk factors of SAH?
- Family history
- Fibromuscular dysplasia
- Coarctation of the aorta
- Congenital polycystic kidney disease
- Moyamoya

O **Assess vital signs**
BP may be elevated
Fever can be a component of SAH

Perform physical and neurologic exam
Check for meningeal irritation by assessing neck stiffness, Kernig's, and Brudzinski's signs
Assess for signs of raised intracranial pressure (ICP) (see p. 20)
Pay close attention of visual fields, pupillary response, ocular movement
- Unilateral dilated pupil with or without other CN3 signs (ptosis, medial rectus palsy) → posterior communicating artery aneurysm at junction of the posterior cerebral artery and internal carotid artery (ICA) compressing CN3
- Visual field cuts → supraclinoid ICA aneurysm compressing CN2
- CN3, CN4, CN5, and CN6 abnormalities → ICA aneurysm in cavernous sinus
- Unilateral or bilateral CN6 palsy → raised ICP from hydrocephalus

Weakness of one or both leg(s)→ aneurysm at anterior cerebral artery
Hemiparesis or aphasia → aneurysm at the first major bifurcation of middle cerebral artery
In approximately 40% of pt, there will be no lateralizing sign.

Grade SAH according to the Botterell, Hunt, and Hess scale
- Grade I — Asymptomatic or with slight headache
- Grade II — Moderate to severe headache, stiff neck, but no lateralizing signs
- Grade III — Drowsy, confusion, and mild focal deficit
- Grade IV — Stupor, obtundation, and obvious focal findings
- Grade V — Coma and decerebrate posturing

Obtain STAT head CT scan without contrast
CT scan is 90% sensitive detecting blood in the first 24 hrs, 80% sensitive at 3 days, and 50% sensitive at 1 wk.
CT is also good for assessing hydrocephalus and other intracranial bleed.

Perform lumbar puncture (LP) if CT results are negative
Usually cerebrospinal fluid (CSF) is grossly bloody within 30 min of SAH, with RBCs reaching 1 million/mm^3.
With small bleed, RBCs may be only a few thousands. LP is the most sensitive at 12 hrs after symptoms start.

To differentiate SAH from traumatic tap, four tubes should be collected with tube 1 and 4 sent for cell count. If RBC count decreases from tube 1 to tube 4 it is more like due to traumatic tap.

Check opening pressure. A high opening pressure is suggestive of SAH.

Xanthochromia (pinkish CSF supernatant) can be seen as early as 2 hours after symptom start and is diagnostic of SAH.

Subarachnoid hemorrhage

Fourth most frequent cerebrovascular accident, after atherothrombosis, embolism, and intracranial hemorrhage.

Annual incidence is approximately 6 to 25 per 100,000 people or 27,000 cases in the U.S.

Peak incidence between 35 and 65 years of age

SAH is mostly caused by non-traumatic rupture of saccular, or "berry," aneurysms.
Arteriovenous malformation (AVM), trauma, and tumors are other causes of SAH.

Saccular aneurysms are outpouchings of arterial vessel covered only by adventitia. Their sizes vary from 2 to 30 mm in diameter. The ones that rupture usually are 10 mm or more.

They arise from arteries of the circle of Willis or its major branches. Approximately 90% are on the anterior half of the circle.

When they rupture, blood under high arterial pressure is forced into the subarachnoid space. The blood in the CSF causes meningeal irritation hence severe headache.

Sometimes the bleeding is very small (sentinel bleed) and self-limited. These may serve as a warning sign of future major rupture.

Bleeding can be severe and causes significant elevation in ICP. Approximately 10% to 15% of pts die before reaching the hospital.

Admit to ICU

Once diagnosis is made, pt needs to be monitored closely

Absolute bed rest with leg squeezers

Fluid hydration to keep slightly hypervolemic

Stool softener to avoid straining

Control BP with IV β-blocker, nitroprusside, or Ca^{2+} channel blocker to keep systolic BP < 150

Pain-relieving medication for headache (this usually will reduce the hypertension)

Start calcium channel blocker

Start nimodipine 60 mg PO Q 4 hrs. It has been shown to reduce the incidence of stroke from vasospasm after SAH.

Obtain brain and brain vasculature imaging

Brain MRI will detect other possible causes of SAH such as AVM and tumors. It also assesses presence of any brain parenchymal damage (e.g., infarct).

MRA and CT angiogram is often used as a screening test for detecting large aneurysms.

Gold standard is to perform carotid and vertebral angiogram (sensitivity ~85%). Drawback is that it is invasive procedure.

Consider transcranial Doppler (TCD)

TCD measures blood flow in intracranial vessels and can detect vasospasms

Consult neurosurgery

To assess and plan for aneurysm surgery or coiling procedure

18 Hydrocephalus

S

Does pt have any symptoms of elevated intracranial pressure (ICP)?
Headache, blurry vision, diplopia, nausea, vomiting

Does the pt have any symptoms of normal pressure hydrocephalus?
Remember the 3 Ws of normal pressure hydrocephalus (NPH)—wet (urinary incontinence), wobbly (gait disturbance), and wacky (dementia)

Is there a history that put pt at risk for developing hydrocephalus?
Subarachnoid hemorrhage, meningitis, head trauma, birth trauma, developmental delay

O

Does pt have any signs of raised ICP?
Decreased level of consciousness, papilledema, bilateral CN6 palsy, sun-setting eyes and vertical gaze palsy, nuchal rigidity
For infants before the cranial sutures fuse, hydrocephalus causes large head. Proper head circumferences are:

- 3 month   35 cm
- 6 month   40 cm
- 9 month   45 cm
- 12 month   50 cm

Obtain head imaging
Head CT is a good way to quickly rule out acute brain pathology
MRI is more sensitive in picking up subtle details and is preferred over CT
Contrast dye should be administered if suspecting tumor or infection
- With communicating hydrocephalus, there is symmetric enlargement of ALL ventricles.
- With non-communicating hydrocephalus, depending on the level of obstruction there will be asymmetric enlargement in the size of lateral, 3rd, and 4th ventricles. For example, if the obstruction is at cerebral aqueduct, the size of 4th ventricle will be normal and sizes of 3rd and lateral ventricles will be large.
- With hydrocephalus ex-vacuo, all ventricles are enlarged as well as the size of fissures and cisterns.
- With normal pressure hydrocephalus, on CT there is ventriculomegaly throughout. On MRI, transependymal edema can be seen surrounding the lateral ventricles.

Obtain cerebrospinal fluid (CSF) sample
In case of communicating hydrocephalus, lumbar puncture can be safely performed. In case of obstructive hydrocephalus, DO NOT perform lumbar puncture because of risk of herniation. CSF should be obtained via neurosurgical means.

Hydrocephalus
hydro = water, cephalus = head
Condition in which too much CSF accumulates within the ventricles
Depending on the type of hydrocephalus, ICP may or may not be elevated

CSF physiology and formation of hydrocephalus
An average adult central nervous system holds approximately 150 cc of CSF with production rate of approximately 500 cc/day.
CSF is produced by choroids plexus in the lateral and third ventricles. It circulates from the brain to the spinal cord and then back to the brain, and finally gets absorbed through the arachnoid villae.

Any imbalance between the rate of production and absorption will result in *communicating hydrocephalus*. Too much CSF production (rare) can be caused by choroids plexus papilloma. Too little CSF absorption can be caused by abnormal CSF content (e.g., cell debris, proteins) clogging up the arachnoid villae. Examples include meningitis, subarachnoid hemorrhage, and CSF carcinomatosis.

Any obstruction in the CSF circulation pathway will result in *non-communicating hydrocephalus*. Examples include brain tumor, intraventricular cysts, cerebral aqueductal stenosis (the most common cause in infants), and brain malformations such as:
- Arnold-Chiari malformations:
  - Type 1: extension of cerebellar tonsils below foramen magnum ± syringomyelia.
  - Type 2: type 1 + displacement of elongated medulla and 4th ventricle into foramen magnum + lumbar meningomyelocele.
  - Type 3: type 2 with more severe cerebellar and brainstem displacement forming a meningoencephalocele.
  - Type 4: hypoplasia of cerebellum and brainstem.
- Dandy-Walker malformation: aplastic cerebellar vermis, cystic dilatation of 4th ventricle

An atrophic or encephalomalacic (tissue loss) brain will have compensatory dilatation of ventricles giving rise to *hydrocephalus ex-vacuo*. It is commonly seen in patients with Alzheimer disease, old stroke, old head trauma, and chronic alcoholism. Intracranial pressure is normal.

When communicating hydrocephalus develops slowly (over months or years), the rate of CSF production and absorption will equilibrate. The CSF pressure is no longer elevated although pt still manifests the cerebral effects of hydrocephalic state. This is *normal pressure hydrocephalus*. It can be seen in pts with remote SAH or meningitis.

Treat hydrocephalus with shunting to relieve raised ICP
For both communicating and non-communicating hydrocephalus, the symptomatic treatment is by shunting.

In emergent cases when pt is showing signs of herniation, ventriculostomy can be done immediately at bedside.

If pt is stable, then permanent shunt can be inserted in the operating room. The shunt has a one-way valve and can redirect CSF to drain into the bloodstream (ventriculoatrial shunt) or peritoneal cavity (ventriculoperitoneal shunt).

Hydrocephalus ex-vacuo does not require any treatment.

Workup and treat the underlying cause
With CSF and MRI the physician should be able to identify whether there is bleed, infection, mass, tumors, malformations. Leave the shunt in the pt until the underlying pathologic process resolves.

For normal pressure hydrocephalus, carefully select shunt candidate
For NPH, treatment is controversial in terms of whether to shunt or not.

Standard is to perform a large volume lumbar puncture (removing > 20–30 cc CSF) to see if there is clinical improvement. Pts who improve are more likely to benefit from shunting.

S **Does pt have any symptoms of raised intracranial pressure (ICP)?**
Common symptoms of elevated ICP include headache, nausea/vomiting, diplopia, visual obscuration, drowsiness, stupor, and coma.

O **Assess ABCs (airway, breathing, and circulation) and vital signs**
Pt may be comatose and unable to protect the airway. Hypopnea and apnea can occur if brainstem is being compressed.

Cushing response is elevated systolic BP (widened pulse pressure) with bradycardia. It is seen when ICP approaches arterial pressure.

Look for signs of elevated ICP
Papilledema, subhyaloid retinal hemorrhage, uni- or bilateral CN6 palsy, restricted upward gaze (sun setting eyes).

Look for signs of herniation
There are four main types of herniation syndromes:
1. Cingulate (a.k.a. subfalcine) herniation occurs when one hemisphere is displaced laterally under the falx. The cingulated lobe is the first to go, along with the anterior cerebral artery, leading to infarction of its territory. Expect to find contralateral leg weakness and urinary incontinence.
2. Uncal herniation occurs when one hemisphere is forced from supratentorial toward infratentorial compartment. The uncus of the displaced medial temporal lobe will compress the ipsilateral CN3, causing pupil dilation and external ocular muscle weakness with the eye deviated laterally (because CN6 is intact). As herniation continues, the midbrain is pushed so that the contralateral cerebral peduncle (*Kernohan's notch*) is compressed, causing hemiparesis on the same side of lesion. The posterior cerebral arteries will be compressed, leading to infarction in the occipital lobes causing blindness.
3. Central herniation occurs when both hemispheres are pushed through the tentorium cerebelli, causing bilateral pupil dilation, followed by quadriparesis and coma.
4. Tonsillar herniation is caused by mass effect in the infratentorial compartment (posterior fossa). The cerebellar tonsils and medulla are pushed through the foramen magnum, causing coma and cardiac/respiratory arrest. The basilar and its feeding branches may be stretched and torn from the downward displacement leading to *Duret hemorrhages* in the pons and midbrain.

Increased Intracranial Pressure
Normal ICP ranges from 6 to 20 mm Hg
The cranium is a *rigid* container that holds three contents: brain, blood, and cerebrospinal fluid (CSF), so that an increase in any one of the three contents will result in elevated ICP.
An increase in volume of any one of the three components must be at the expense of the other two, a relationship known as the Monro-Kellie doctrine.
Of the three intracranial components, the brain is the least compressible. The CSF compartment can divert CSF into the spinal space, and the vascular space can shrink by vasoconstriction. However, the brain is not compressible and once the CSF and vascular buffer have been exhausted, the brain will displace (herniate) from one dural space to the other.
When ICP reaches critical point, cerebral blood flow will be cut off and will produce widespread ischemia (cerebral perfusion pressure [CPP] = mean arterial pressure [MAP] − ICP)

Mechanisms generating elevated ICP:
1. Mass lesion: can be either axial (inside the brain, e.g., brain tumor, infarction with edema, hematoma, contusion, abscess) or extra-axial (outside of brain, e.g., meningioma, subdural/epidural hematomas)
2. Generalized brain swelling: anoxic brain injury, hypertensive encephalopathy, Reye syndrome (unexplained cerebral edema and liver failure following viral illness), acute liver failure
3. Increase in venous pressure: cerebral venous thrombosis, obstruction of jugular or superior mediastinal veins
4. CSF flow obstruction or volume expansion: Both obstructive and non-obstructive hydrocephalus can cause ↑ ICP

P Stabilize pt first
If pt is comatose or apneic, this will necessitate intubation to protect the airway and prevent hypoxia. Obtain baseline ABG. Keep O_2 saturation > 93%.

Maintain blood pressure. Remember CPP = MAP − ICP. Use isotonic fluid such as normal saline or lactated Ringer. Avoid hypotonic fluids, which can worsen cerebral edema. Keep fluid in & out balanced or slightly negative.

Keep the head of the bed elevated approximately 30 degrees to lower ICP as well as the risk of aspiration.

Treat fever aggressively with antipyretics and cooling measures. Hyperthermia increases neuronal damage.

Agitation and excessive movement will worsen ICP. Use sedatives if necessary.

Phenobarbital can reduce cerebral metabolic activity and may help areas that have decreased cerebral perfusion to survive.

If patient is showing signs of herniation
Intubate immediately and hyperventilate to $PaCO_2$ < 25

The receptors in the brain sense the drop in $PaCO_2$ and tell the intracranial vessels to constrict, thereby decrease blood volume and ICP. The effect is immediate (within seconds to minutes) but is not long lasting (hours).

Start mannitol 0.5 to 1 g/kg IV bolus, then 25 g IV Q 6 hrs for 3 to 5 days

Monitor Na level and serum osmolarity. Hold if Na > 150 or osmolarity > 310

Mannitol works by sucking extravascular (brain) water into intravascular space and then excreting it through kidney. The brain volume decreases.

Mannitol works within hours and the effect lasts for days.

Consult neurosurgery
Ventriculostomy allows CSF to drain outside and create more rooms to relieve pressure.

Craniotomy will allow brain to expand against no pressure. It is the most drastic but effective measure to relieve elevated pressure. The skull can be placed back at later time.

Determine the etiology causing raised ICP and treat the underlying cause
Head CT without contrast if stroke, hemorrhage, trauma, subarachnoid hemorrhage are suspected.

Head CT with contrast or MRI if tumor, abscess, or meningitis are suspected.

S **Does the pt have any neurologic symptoms?**
Most pts present in one of the following ways:
- Seizure
- Headache (very common with arteriovenous malformation [AVM], can be migraine-like)
- Hemorrhage
- Focal neurologic deficit (e.g., numbness, weakness)
- Asymptomatic, lesion is found incidentally

What is the age of the pt?
Vascular malformations are congenital and present at birth. The majority become symptomatic in early adulthood. So when a young pt presents with hemorrhage or seizure, vascular malformation should always be in the differential diagnosis.

Obtain detailed family history including seizure and neurologic symptoms
Some vascular malformations are hereditary. The family member might not have a known diagnosis but may have a history of neurologic symptoms.

 Perform general and neurologic exam
Check for systolic bruit over the carotid artery, mastoid process, and eyeballs. If present in a young pt, it is almost pathognomic of an AVM.
In young children with very large AVM, the arteriovenous shunting may cause high-output cardiac failure.

Obtain and review brain and vascular imaging
If pt presents acutely, get CT to quickly rule out an acute bleed.
MRI of brain with contrast is preferred in a non-urgent setting.
Cerebral angiogram is required for hemodynamic assessment, which is essential for planning surgery.

 Vascular malformations
The four major types of vascular malformations are, in order of frequency, venous malformation, AVM, cavernous hemangioma, and telangiectasia. They are listed below in order of clinical importance.

1. Arteriovenous malformation
AVMs are congenital lesions composed of a complex tangle of arteries and veins directly connected without an intervening capillary network. The venous blood is arteriolized and under higher than normal pressure.
Onset of symptoms is most common between 10 and 30 years old.
In almost 50% of pts, the first presentation is a cerebral subarachnoid hemorrhage.
In the other 50% of pts, the first presentation is seizure, headache, or focal neurologic deficit.
Hemorrhage from AVM represents 2% of all strokes.

2. Cavernous malformation
A.k.a., cavernous hemangioma, cavernous angioma, cavernoma
They are like "blood sponges," made up of variable sized vascular spaces; when looked under microscope, appears to be caves, hence the name "cavernous."
Unlike AVM, there's no brain tissue between these vascular spaces.
The blood flow within these sinusoids is slow and stagnant with thrombosis in various stages of organization.
Onset of symptoms is usually between 20 and 50 years of age.
Approximately 50% of pts present with seizure as first presentation; 40% present with hemorrhage or focal neurologic symptoms; 10% present with headache.

Some cavernous malformations are hereditary (particularly in Hispanics) and some are sporadic. Lesions can be solitary or multiple.

3. Venous malformation (venous angioma)
They are made of abnormally dilated veins that coalesce together to form a large vein ("caput medusae") and drain into ventricular or cortical surface.
Although they are congenital, they may enlarge with time.
They may be associated with cavernous malformation.
They are benign lesions and rarely bleed. Most pts are asymptomatic and diagnosis is made incidentally.

4. Capillary telangiectasia
They are small lesions made up of tiny capillary vessels with normal brain tissue in between. There are no obviously dilated feeding arteries.
Pts with telangiectasia are rarely symptomatic. Most are found incidentally during autopsy.

Treat the acute symptoms first
Refer to the notes on ICH, SAH, seizure, and headache.

Decide to treat or not to treat and how to treat
The decision is difficult. One must consider pt's age, symptom, and location of malformation. Knowledge of the natural history of these lesions is also very important.

1. AVM
The rate of hemorrhage in untreated pts is 2% to 4% per year. In other words, if left untreated approximately 50% of pt will experience hemorrhage after 15 years. Most physicians recommend treating AVMs.

The options include surgical excision, endovascular embolization, and radiosurgery.

2. CM
The rate of hemorrhage is approximately 1.5% per lesion per year. After the first bleed, risk increases to 4.5% per year.
Most neurologists and neurosurgeons agree that indications for surgery include:
- Recurrent overt hemorrhage
- Medically intractable seizure
- Severe or progressive neurologic symptoms

Asymptomatic lesions need not be resected.
Best treatment is by surgical excision. Radiosurgery is not recommended at present.

3. Venous malformation and telangiectasia
These are usually benign and do not require treatment.

Traumatic Brain Injury

S **Obtain details on mechanism of injury and associated symptoms**
Fall, motor vehicle accident, assault, penetrating wound.
Ask about loss of consciousness (LOC), amnesia, seizures, and symptoms of ↑ intracranial pressure (ICP).

O **Assess vital signs**
Hypertension and bradycardia (Cushing's response) may indicate ↑ ICP. Observe pattern of breathing. Cheyne-Stokes (alternating periods of hyperventilation [HV] and apnea) is seen in bilateral deep brain injury or uncal herniation. Ataxic respiration suggests medullary involvement. Apneustic respiration (prolonged inspiration) or neurogenic HV can be seen in pontine lesions.
Neurogenic shock is seen in cervical cord injuries. The sympathetic chain is interrupted and pt has hypotension, bradycardia, normal central venous pressure (CVP), and normal hematocrit (Hct). This needs to be differentiated from hypovolemic shock which has hypotension, tachycardia, low CVP, and low Hct.
Hypothermia and hyperthermia may suggest hypothalamic dysfunction.

Perform general physical
Palpate the skull for depressed skull fracture or scalp swelling.
Battle and raccoon signs indicate basilar skull fracture.
Rhinorrhea or otorrhea may be due to cerebrospinal fluid (CSF) leak with basilar skull fracture. Normal nasal or ear discharges are without glucose and it can be distinguished from CSF easily with a glucose dipstick test.
Check for neck stiffness, which indicates the presence of subarachnoid hemorrhage. Before turning the neck, make sure pt is cleared for C-spine injury.
Auscultate and palpate carotid arteries for sign of occlusion, which is seen with carotid dissection in neck injury.
Auscultate heart and lung for hemopericardium and pneumo/hemothorax.
Examine abdomen for ruptured spleen, liver, kidney, and bladder.

Perform a complete neurologic exam
Begin with Glasgow coma scale (GCS) (see appendix).
For the best motor response part in GCS: Decorticate posture (arms flexed and legs extended) signifies lesion between the cortex and red nucleus in midbrain.
Decerebrate posture (arms and legs extended) indicate lesion between red nucleus and vestibular nuclei in upper medulla. Absence of motor response indicates lesion in lower medulla or spinal cord.
Carefully examine pupil. Unilateral fixed and dilated pupil indicates ipsilateral uncal herniation. Unilateral miosis and ptosis suggest Horner's syndrome from cervicothoracic spinal cord, brachial plexus, or carotid artery injury. Bilateral small pupils can be seen in drug intoxication or pontine injury. Afferent pupillary defect is seen in optic nerve or retinal injury.
Observe extraocular muscles. Horizontal gaze palsy is seen in lesions affecting either pontine gaze center or frontal eye field. If pt is comatose, perform Doll's eye test. If patient is comatose, but on C-spine precaution, perform cold caloric test.

Send off routine labs
Chemistry, CBC with differential, PT, PTT, creatine kinase, ABG, toxicology screen, EtOH level, CXR

Obtain head CT with bone window
CT scan is good for skull fracture; intracranial hemorrhage; subdural, epidural hematoma; and subarachnoid hemorrhage.

Cerebral edema and diffuse axonal injury may be missed on a CT scan, especially in early stages. MRI is more sensitive.

Traumatic brain injury
Very common condition seen across emergency departments, estimated at 200 cases per 100,000 people. Male:female is 2:1. More common in people < 35 years of age.
Concussion is the most minor brain injury. Pt has LOC and mild amnesia. By definition, no structural brain injury is seen. Postconcussive syndrome constitutes of persistent headache, nausea, decreased concentration, poor memory, insomnia, and depression.
Contusion is an area of hemorrhagic necrosis (brain bruise) following a nonpenetrating blow to head. Most common sites are subfrontal and anterior temporal lobes due to the irregular bony contours of anterior and middle cranial fossa. Contusion at site of impact is called coup injury and happens when the head is struck while still. Contusion at opposite side of head from site of impact is called contra-coup injury and happens when head was moving and hit a stationary object.
Brain lacerations are caused by penetrating injuries such as bullets and depressed skull fracture. There is higher chance for seizures and infections.
Diffuse axonal injury is caused by shearing forces that damage axons during acceleration and deceleration. Pt often is comatose or has severe focal deficits without evidence of hematoma and infarction on CT. Recovery is usually limited.
Epidural hematoma is caused by rupture of *middle meningeal artery* (less often veins) between outer surface of dura matter and inner table of skull. Pt may be lucid initially but deteriorates within minutes to hours to becoming comatose and dead. On CT, an epidural hematoma is lenticular shaped and *does not cross suture lines*.
Subdural hematoma is caused by rupture of *bridging veins* between the inner dura and arachnoid. They usually occur over cerebral convexities, are bilateral in 15% of cases, and *cross suture lines*. Clinical course can be acute (minutes to hours), subacute (days), or chronic (weeks to months).

Determine severity of the injury
Take into account GCS score and clinical picture. Pt with concussion can be discharged home. Pts with moderate to severe traumatic brain injuries (TBIs) need to be admitted.

Consult neurosurgery
Indications for surgery include open skull fracture or >1 cm depressed skull fracture, penetrating injury requiring debridement, >30 cc intra-axial hematoma, extra-axial hematoma with midline shift > 5 mm, and posterior fossa hematomas.
Invasive ICP monitor is also indicated when increased ICP is encountered.

Manage ICP
This is the major part of care for TBI. Pts with moderate to severe TBI often have diffuse cerebral edema, hemorrhages, and infarcts that will cause ↑ ICP and herniation syndrome. (See ICP management, p. 20.)

Supportive medical care
Syndrome of inappropriate antidiuretic hormone secretion is seen commonly in brain injuries and may cause further brain swelling if not treated. Be careful not to correct hyponatremia too rapidly, which will cause central pontine myelinolysis.
Start anticonvulsants if pt has seizure. The use of anti-epileptic drugs will prevent patient from having seizures from the acute TBI. It does not alter the long-term development of post-traumatic epilepsy (recurrent seizures).
Obtain EEG and evoked potential for prognosis.

III
Seizures

Are there any risk factors for seizure?
- History of head trauma
- Family history of seizure
- Mental retardation and developmental delay
- History of meningitis or encephalitis
- History of febrile convulsion

Is there any provoking factor?
Drugs (EtOH, cocaine), lack of sleep, fever, head trauma

Was there aura before seizure onset?
Presence of aura indicates partial onset seizure. Common auras include:
- Déjà vu
- GI sensation
- Visual changes
- Hallucinations
- Funny taste or smell

Ask for description of seizure
It is helpful to ask a witness because most pts are amnesic during the event.
Ask how the seizure started. Was pt jerking one or both sides? Was there gaze deviation during the seizure?
Ask about tongue biting and urinary incontinence. These indicate a generalized seizure.
Ask about postictal state. Was there focality during postictal state, e.g., hemiparesis (Todd's paralysis), gaze deviation? These are seen in partial onset seizures.

Perform a general and neurologic exam
Note any asymmetric weakness
Check for spontaneous smile. Asymmetry may suggest temporal lobe lesion.

Review pertinent laboratory data
CBC, chemistry panel, liver and thyroid function tests, and toxicology screen

Obtain head imaging
Most pts with first-time seizure present to the emergency department. Head CT should be obtained and is sensitive to rule out most acute issues.
For pts with partial-onset seizure with negative results on CT, MRI of the brain with thin cuts through medial temporal lobes with/without contrast should be obtained.

Consider EEG
Pts without obvious provoking factors should undergo screening EEG. A normal EEG does not rule out seizure. However, an abnormal EEG with spikes and sharp waves is diagnostic of seizure disorder.

Consider lumbar puncture (LP)
LP is indicated if infection is suspected.

Seizure
An intermittent derangement of the nervous system due to an excessive and disorderly discharge of cerebral nervous tissue.
Seizure is a sign, not a diagnosis. It is the manifestation of an underlying central nervous or systemic medical illness.
If seizure becomes recurrent, then it is called epilepsy.
Seizure is common. It is estimated 1% of U.S. population will have seizure by age of 20.

Is the episode in question really a seizure?
This is the most important question the neurologist has to answer. Often it is difficult to answer.

Conditions that might mimic a seizure episode include:
- Syncope
- Transient ischemic attack
- Complicated migraine
- Panic attack
- Hypoglycemia
- Sleep disorders such as narcolepsy
- Pseudoseizure (a.k.a. psychogenic seizure, nonepileptic seizure)

One has to take into account the history, exam, age of pt, and presence of other concurrent medical conditions, then come up with an answer.

Factors that support diagnosis of seizure include presence of aura, stereotypical episodes, injuries (tongue laceration on the sides, falls, burns), abnormal neurologic exam, EEG, and MRI.

Pelvic thrusting, side-to-side head shaking, tongue biting at the tip, and eyes closing during event are more consistent with psychogenic seizure.

Postictal confusion or amnesia are found in either seizure or syncope. Todd's paralysis is seen only in seizure. If the paralysis lasts more than 24 hrs, stroke has to be ruled out.

Decide whether to start pt on medication

Once the seizure is diagnosed, next step is to assess the risk of having recurrent seizure.

If the seizure is provoked (i.e., febrile seizure, EtOH, sleep deprivation), there is no need to treat with anti-epileptic medication.

If the seizure is unprovoked, then use clinical judgment to decide. If there is clear evidence supporting increased chance of having recurrent seizures (e.g., abnormal MRI or EEG) then patient should be treated.

Educate pt about seizure

If the seizure is non-provoked and all test results are negative, the chance of having a second seizure is approximately 25% over next 2 yrs.

If the seizure is provoked, the physician must stress the importance of avoiding those provoking factors, such as EtOH, cocaine, sleep deprivation.

Advise pt to avoid doing things that might cause harm if second seizure occurs. Examples include driving motor vehicles, swimming alone, climbing ladders, and operating heavy machinery.

Report case to state's department of motor vehicles

It is the responsibility of the treating physician to report any case of loss of consciousness to the department of motor vehicle.

The government, not the physician, makes the decision whether or not to suspend the license. Regulation varies from state to state, but most pts get their license back if seizure does not recur (with or without treatment) after few months.

The physician is liable for not reporting if the pt has a vehicular accident injuring self or other people.

Epilepsy

S **Inquire about seizure control?**
Ask about the frequency of seizure and date of the last episode. Ask pts to record seizures on a seizure calendar. The seizure frequency serves as a monitor for efficacy of treatment.

What is the seizure semiology?
Ask about auras, description of seizure, and presence of postictal state (see Seizure p. 28).

What antiepileptic drugs is the pt taking and has taken?
There is a variety of seizure medications. Knowing what medication has worked or failed in the past will be very helpful.
Ask about compliance because noncompliance is the most common reason for failure of therapy.

Does the pt experience any side effects from the anti-epileptic drugs (AED)?
The most common seizure medications and their side effects:
- Phenytoin (PHT): gingival hyperplasia, Stevens-Johnson, hepatitis, ataxia
- Carbamazepine (CBZ): aplastic anemia, Stevens-Johnson, ↓ Na, ataxia
- Oxcarbazepine (OXC): same as CBZ, but better tolerated in general
- Valproic acid (VPA): hepatitis, pancreatitis, ↓ platelet count, rash, weight gain
- Phenobarbital (PB): hepatitis, rash, hyperactivity in children, ↓ IQ
- Topiramate (TPM): nephrolithiasis, ↓ weight, oligohidrosis, glaucoma, ↓ IQ
- Levetiracetam (LEV): psychosis, agitation, emotional lability
- Zonisamide (ZNS): same as topiramate
- Gabapentin (GBP): dizziness, somnolence
- Lamotrigine (LTG): Stevens-Johnson, dizziness
- Vigabatrin (VGB): Visual field constriction

O **Perform a general and neurologic exam**
Pay attention to signs of toxicity from AEDs, especially gingival hyperplasia, nystagmus, ataxia, and skin rashes. Observe pt's gait.

Order and review pertinent laboratory data
PHT, CBZ, VPA, and PB levels can be monitored in serum. Levels serve as compliance indicator. Levels can also be affected by drug interactions.
Periodically monitor liver function tests, especially with phenytoin and valproate.
For pts taking CBZ and OXC, monitor CBC and Na level.

Obtain EEG
EEG should be performed on all pts with epilepsy. EEG can determine the seizure type (partial vs. generalized) and screen for epilepsy syndromes (e.g., 3-Hz spike-wave in absence, hypsarrhythmia in infantile spasm).
Also helpful in deciding whether or not to discontinue AED after seizure has been controlled for a time.

Consider head imaging
If the seizure type is primary generalized (as indicated by EEG), then there is no need to perform head imaging.
If the seizure type is partial onset with/without secondary generalization, MRI of brain with thin coronal cuts through temporal lobes with/without contrast is indicated. MR spectroscopy may also be helpful in identifying mesial temporal sclerosis.

Epilepsy
Defined as two or more recurrent seizures.
Prevalence is approximately 4.7/1000 persons. The incidence is the greatest for the very young (<15 y/o) and very old (>65 y/o).
Major causes of epilepsy include structural brain lesions (congenital malformations, tumors, strokes), previous brain injuries (head trauma, meningitis), and idiopathic.
When epilepsy has distinctive features such as age onset, seizure symptoms, disease progression, and EEG/MRI patterns, it falls into the category of *epilepsy syndromes*. (See p. 30.) They are often, but not always, genetic.

Maximize medical control
The goal of epilepsy therapy is to achieve as few seizures as possible while minimizing side effects from medications.
If the seizure is not under control, first rule out these possibilities
- Pt is not compliant with medication.
- The drug level is subtherapeutic.
- Pt is not getting the correct medication for the seizure type.
  - PHT, CBZ, PB work only for partial-onset seizure, not primary generalized seizure.

Add second or third AEDs, if necessary
- When adding additional AED, take into account drug interaction and side effects.
- For example, mixing phenytoin (a P-450 inducer) and valproic acid (P-450 inhibitor) will have unpredictable drug interactions and the levels may become either subtherapeutic or toxic.

Consider surgical options
If the seizure remains intractable despite being on multiple therapeutic medications, surgical options can be considered. The options include vagal nerve stimulator (VNS), lesionectomy, temporal lobectomy, hemispherectomy, corpus callosotomy, and subpial transection. VNS and temporal lobectomy are the most common types of surgery performed.
VNS is a small metallic device implanted in the anterior subcutaneous chest.
It has a wire that connects to the vagus nerve.
The device sends an electrical signal to vagus nerve at determined rate and has an effect of decreasing seizure frequency.
When pt feels seizure is coming or when family member sees pt is having a seizure, he or she can briefly turn up the device with an external magnet, thus abolish the seizure. Approximately 45% VNS pts will have > 50% reduction in seizures.
Temporal lobectomy is performed on pts with demonstrable lesions (both on MRI and EEG) in one of the temporal lobes.
A Wada test is done before surgery to ensure pt will not have severe language or memory deficit after the surgery.
The lesion can be resected either by conventional surgery or radiosurgery using a gamma knife.

Approximately 75% of pts have complete resolution of epilepsy after the surgery. Most will have significant reduction in seizure frequency.

32 Status Epilepticus

How long has the seizure been going on?
The majority of seizures resolve spontaneously within 1 to 2 min. If the seizure has been going on for > 10 min, then pt is in status epilepticus.
Alternatively, pt is in status epilepticus (SE) if he/she has multiple short seizures > 30 min apart without regaining baseline mental status.

Quickly review the history from the family or medical chart
Is the pt a known epileptic? If yes, on what medication? Is the pt compliant with treatment?
Any obvious cause of seizure? For example, stroke, intracranial hemorrhage, subarachnoid hemorrhage, tumor?
Review medication list

Assess vital signs
Fever, hypertension, shock, and arrhythmia are commonly seen in SE.

Perform quick physical and neurologic exam
Check for evidence of stroke with asymmetric pupil, gaze deviation, and hemiparesis. Note that after focal seizures, the seizure focus may be hypoactive and may appear like a stroke (Todd's paralysis).
Signs of drug abuse: smell of EtOH, pinpoint pupils, and needle tracks.
Neck stiffness and fever suggest meningitis or subarachnoid hemorrhage.
Look for signs of head injury. Examine the scalp and skull.

Send routine labs
Chem panel; glucose, Ca, Mg, CBC, urinalysis, PT, PTT, toxicology screen, and AED levels

Obtain STAT EEG
The only way to rule out subclinical status is by obtaining an EEG.

Obtain STAT head CT
Especially if pt does not have obvious cause of having seizure.

Consider lumbar puncture
If infection, vasculitis, or subarachnoid hemorrhage is suspected.

Status Epilepticus
Definition: continuous seizure activity lasting more than 10 min or intermittent seizure activity lasting more than 30 min during which consciousness is not regained.
In the U.S., the annual incidence of SE is 150,000 to 200,000 with 26% mortality rate. Study has shown the longer the duration of SE, the higher the mortality.
Etiologies of SE, from most to least common, include:

1. Discontinuation of AED
2. Stroke
3. Alcohol withdrawal
4. Idiopathic
5. Anoxia
6. Intracranial hemorrhage
7. Meningitis or encephalitis
8. Tumor
9. Trauma
10. Drugs such as cocaine, theophylline, isoniazid

Complications of SE include rising temperature, acidosis, hypertension and hypotension, hypoxia, hypercarbia, hyperkalemia, hypoglycemia, arrhythmia, pulmonary edema, aspiration pneumonia, and renal failure from myoglobinuria or acute tubular necrosis.

Stabilize pt
Turn pt on the side to prevent aspiration. Establish oral airway.
Intubate if pt hypoxic or unable to protect airway.
Hypotension should be addressed with normal saline infusion and/or pressors.

Start benzodiazepine
Give lorazepam (Ativan) 0.1 mg/kg by IV push at rate of 2 mg/min
Alternatively, diazepam (Valium) may be used at 2 mg/min until seizure stops or a total of 20 mg has been given.
Benzodiazepine works by binding to GABA receptors in the brain, increases the frequency of channel opening and thus enhances GABAergic inhibition of CNS.

Start phenytoin or fosphenytoin
Load phenytoin 20 mg/kg IV at infusion rate of 50 mg/min, and then continue at 100 mg IV Q 8 hrs. Side effects include hypotension, arrhythmia, respiratory depression, and thrombophlebitis.
Fosphenytoin is a water-soluble pro-drug of phenytoin. It is administered at the same dose as phenytoin but at faster rate of 150 mg/min. It can also be given IM when IV access is not available. It causes fewer side effects than phenytoin. If available, it is preferred over phenytoin.
Additional dose of 5 mg/kg can be given if seizure continues.

If seizure continues, intubate pt and start phenobarbital or valproic acid
Before starting phenobarbital, endotracheal tube should be inserted and O_2 administered due to phenobarbital's side effect of respiratory depression.
Load with phenobarbital 20 mg/kg IV at rate of 100 mg/min.
Can give additional 5–10 mg/kg if seizure continues after loading dose
Alternatively, load valproic acid 20 mg/kg IV at rate of 3 mg/kg/min. Valproic acid does not cause respiratory and cardiovascular depression.

If seizure continues, start anesthesia with midazolam or propofol
Midazolam 0.2 mg/kg loading dose followed by an infusion of 0.1–0.4 mg/kg/hr as determined by clinical and EEG monitoring
Propofol 2 mg/kg loading dose followed by IV drip of 2–8 mg/kg/hr
Both medications cause hypotension and frequently pressors are needed to maintain BP

If seizure continues, start pentobarbital
Pentobarbital load 10–15 mg/kg IV over 1 hr, followed by 0.5–1 mg/kg/hr.
Pentobarbital is one of the most potent seizure medications. It will almost always stop seizure by inducing coma, suppressing all brain activity.
It is reserved for last resort because it can cause severe hypotension and postinfusion weakness, which may delay weaning from ventilatory support.

After seizure stops, obtain STAT EEG
Although clinical generalized convulsion stops, pt may still have subclinical electrical status. The only way to find that out is by EEG monitoring.
Proceed in the previous algorithm if electrical status continues.

Perform secondary survey
SE should be treated before sending pt to x-ray, CT, or MRI. After the seizure has stopped both clinically and on EEG, the physician should determine the underlying cause of SE and treat.

Epilepsy Syndromes

S **Obtain detailed description of seizures**

Epilepsy syndromes are a group of diseases with distinctive age of onset/offset, seizure symptoms, exam findings, EEG, and neuroimaging findings. It is important to identify these pts because treatments and prognosis are different.

Seizure symptom can be characterized as follows:
- Tonic: stiffening of body, upward deviation of eyes
- Clonic: rhythmic jerking of arms and legs
- Tonic-clonic: initial tonic followed by clonic phase
- Atonic: brief loss of muscle tone and consciousness, causing abrupt falls
- Absence: sudden and brief blank stare with immediate return to baseline
- Atypical absence: like absence but has gradual onset and lasts > 10 seconds
- Myoclonic: sudden muscle jerks

Most epilepsy syndromes are seen in pediatric population. Obtain birth and developmental history, the age of disease onset, and associated neurologic symptoms.

 Perform complete general and neurologic exam

Presence of cerebral palsy or mental retardation makes West syndrome and Lennox-Gastaut syndrome high in differential diagnosis.

Examine skin for evidence of tuberous sclerosis or neurofibromatosis.

Obtain EEG

EEG is the most important diagnostic tool in epilepsy syndromes. A single negative EEG does not rule out epilepsy. As the number of times that EEG is performed increases, so does the sensitivity of diagnosing epilepsy.

The goal of EEG is to evaluate the interictal (between seizures) background brain activity and to capture the abnormal ictal activity. Several maneuvers are performed to increase the yield. They include photic stimulation, hyperventilation, sleep deprivation, and sleep induction.

Consider brain imaging

Getting MRI or CT in pediatric group is a major procedure often requiring anesthesia; therefore, do not inadvertently order these studies. In most cases, the diagnosis of epilepsy syndromes does not require any imaging.

 Selected Epilepsy Syndromes

West Syndrome (a.k.a., infantile spasms [IS]): Onset is usually in pts < 1 year old. Defined as a triad of IS, mental retardation, and interictal EEG pattern of hypsarrhythmia (very high-voltage slow waves with superimposed multifocal spike and waves). IS are sudden and brief (5 to 10 seconds) tonic contractions involving trunk and limb flexors and/or extensors. They often occur in clusters. Causes can be from any type of brain injury (e.g., stroke, hypoxia, hemorrhage) or can be idiopathic. As pts grow older, the disease may develop into Lennox Gastaut syndrome.

Benign rolandic epilepsy (BRE): Onset is at 5 to 9 years of age, with an autosomal dominant inheritance. Normal development. Pt has nocturnal focal motor seizures (e.g., unilateral face, arm, or leg jerking) with secondary generalization (spread to entire body with loss of consciousness [LOC]). EEG, especially during sleep, shows high-voltage spikes in contralateral lower rolandic or centrotemporal area. Seizures are easy to treat and disappear by adolescence.

Benign occipital epilepsy (BOE): Similar to BRE, but the spikes are in occipital area and seizures start with visual symptoms (hallucination, blindness).

Lennox Gastaut syndrome (LGS): Onset is usually 2 to 6 years of age. Cause can be idiopathic or associated with severe brain insult (stroke, hypoxia, malformation). Characterized by triad of multiple seizure types (tonic, atonic, absence, myoclonic, generalized tonic-clonic [GTC]), mental retardation or regression, and abnormal interictal EEG with generalized slow (1.5 to 2 Hz) spike-and-wave. Prognosis is poor with lifelong epilepsy that is difficult to control.

Juvenile myoclonic epilepsy (JME): Onset is during adolescence and early 20s. Seizures occur in the morning shortly after awakening, especially with sleep deprivation, EtOH, and stress. Seizures are generalized and can be myoclonic (without LOC), GTC, or absence. EEG characteristically shows bursts of 4 to 6 Hz irregular polyspike-and-waves. Intelligence is not affected. Pt likely will have lifelong seizures that are easily controlled with medication.

Absence seizures: Onset between 4 and 11 years of age. Seizure is generalized, sudden, and brief (seconds). Pt will have abrupt interruption of consciousness, halt what he/she is doing, appears to have blank stare, and then resume the activity. Pts do not fall. There may be hundreds of spells per day. The spells are so brief they may go unnoticed by others and pt's disease may manifest as deterioration in schoolwork. EEG shows ictal 3-Hz spike-and-wave discharge often enhanced by hyperventilation. Absence goes away by adolescence but may be replaced by other generalized epilepsy.

Febrile seizure: Occurs between 6 months to 5 years of age. Generalized motor seizures caused by fever from illnesses not related to CNS (e.g., flu, pneumonia, otitis media). EEG is normal. This condition is benign and has strong genetic component. Risk of developing epilepsy is only slightly greater than that in the general population. No medication is needed.

Landau Kleffner syndrome (acquired epileptic aphasia): Onset 4 to 7 years of age. Pts progressively lose language ability along with development of seizures of GTC or myoclonic type. Prognosis varies with some pts regain most of language function. Seizures are usually easy to control.

Reflex epilepsy: Onset ranges from childhood to early adulthood. Seizures are of GTC or myoclonic type and are induced by external stimuli with visual (light flashing) being the most common but auditory, olfactory, or internal mental process (reading, doing math) are possible. EEG with photic stimulation often elicits the underlying EEG abnormality.

P **Identify the syndrome and start appropriate treatment**
Benign seizures such as febrile seizure, BRE, and BOE do not require treatment. The disease is self-limited and pts will outgrow them.
For absence seizure, valproic acid or ethosuximide are the drugs of choice.
Carbamazepine and phenytoin may worsen the seizure.
For JME, valproic acid is the first choice.
For IS, start with ACTH or corticosteroid. Clonazepam may be added.
For LGS, seizures are usually difficult to control and require multiple anti-epileptic drugs.
Ketogenic diet may be beneficial in controlling intractable epilepsy.
Vagal nerve stimulator may be considered.
Corpus callosotomy may be effective in reducing generalized seizures (because the connection between the two hemispheres is resected) and drop attacks. It is palliative only. Pt will continue to have partial seizures.

How old is the pt?
The pts in this group of epilepsy are mostly young adults to adults. For younger pts, consider the diagnosis of epilepsy syndromes first.

Inquire about the details of seizure episode
Refer to history taking section of General Epilepsy (p. 30).
Ask whether the consciousness was impaired (i.e., was pt aware of or remember what was going on at the time of event?).
If consciousness was not impaired, then the seizure is simple partial seizure.
If consciousness was impaired, then it is complex partial seizure.
If the pt goes into a generalized convulsion (i.e., with bilateral tonic-clonic movement, tongue biting, urinary incontinence), then it's called simple or complex partial seizure with secondary generalization.

Perform a complete general and neurologic exam
Most pts with epilepsy will have a normal exam.

Obtain EEG
Pts with localization related epilepsies often have abnormal discharges (spikes or sharp waves) or focal slowing in the abnormal area.

Order an MRI of brain with thin cuts through temporal lobes with/without contrast
Temporal lobe seizures are the most common and most likely to benefit from surgical resection.

Temporal lobe epilepsy
Evolutionarily the temporal lobe is the oldest part of the brain and is also the most epileptogenic. It carries the most primitive senses such as sexual drive, hunger, fear, and smell.
The initial symptom of temporal lobe epilepsy (TLE) is based on where the seizure originates.
- Medial basal (amygdala-hippocampal): increasing epigastric discomfort, autonomic signs such as pallor, flushing, mydriasis, irregular respiration, abdominal borborygmi, eructation, fearful, olfactory, and gustatory auras.
- Lateral (neocortical): auditory and/or visual sensory hallucination/distortion, psychic dreamy states, and aphasias.

Toward the latter phase of seizure motor components occur and consist of automatisms such as lip smacking, chewing, fumbling of hands, and shuffling of feet.
The seizure can stop there and pt goes into postictal state or can continue to secondarily generalize to both hemispheres.
The most common cause of TLE is hippocampal sclerosis (a.k.a., mesiotemporal sclerosis), which may be caused by previous head trauma, hypoxic injury, recurrent seizures. Other causes of TLE include post encephalitis, vascular malformation, tumors, and trauma.

Frontal lobe epilepsies
Often misdiagnosed as psychogenic episodes.
Frontal lobe epilepsy seizures are usually brief, stereotyped, occur during sleep, complex partial with little or no postictal confusion, rapid secondary generalization, prominent motor manifestation, frequent complex gestural automatisms at onset, frequent falling if charges are bilateral.
Most common causes include congenital causes such as cortical dysgenesis, gliosis, or vascular malformations; neoplasms; head trauma; infections; and anoxia.

Parietal lobe epilepsy

Functions of the parietal lobe include sensory, visual-spatial construction.
Parietal lobe epilepsy is often sensory at onset (tingling, electricity, crawling, stiffness, cold, or pain) with variable secondary generalization.
Visual hallucinations of parietal origin are usually structured.
Postictally, one may find asomatognosia, cortical sensory deficits, spatial disorientation, and dyscalculia.
Most common causes include vascular malformations, tumors, and trauma.

Occipital lobe epilepsy

Occipital lobe carries visual functions.
Occipital lobe epilepsy usually involves eye movements, head turning, and/or visual hallucinations. The hallucinations from the anterior occipital lobe tend to generate more structured images or image distortions such as macropsia or micropsia. The hallucinations from the posterior occipital lobe tend to be unstructured lights, colors, and flashes.
Most common causes include trauma, drugs (especially immunosuppressants), and hypertensive crisis.

P Treat with anti-convulsants

All these disorders are partial seizures and therefore all anti-epileptic drugs will work on them. The choice of medication varies individually.

Plan for epilepsy surgery

Surgery can be curative if the seizure focus is removed.
To demonstrate that all seizures come from a single place, prolonged EEG (3 to 7 days) is required. The pt is admitted to the hospital and attached to a video EEG machine. The medications are discontinued with intention to provoke as many seizures as possible. The seizures are then analyzed on the EEG and video.
Sometimes scalp EEG is not adequate and stereotactically placed depth electrode or subdural grid EEG is needed to localize the seizure focus.
If all the seizures arise from a single focus, then pt is a surgical candidate.
Before lobectomy can be done, a Wada test (named after neurologist John Wada) is done by first injecting a short-acting anesthetic (e.g., amobarbital or Brevital) into a carotid artery. The anesthetic will temporarily shut down one hemisphere. A set of words, pictures, shapes are shown and read to the pt. After the anesthetic effect is gone (usually 5 to 10 min), pt is asked to recall the items shown during the test. The test is then repeated with anesthesia injected to the other hemisphere.
The Wada test will establish which hemisphere has dominant language and memory functions and whether resection is feasible without causing significant intellectual deficit.
If pt passes the Wada test, surgery can then be scheduled. Temporal lobectomy is the most frequently performed procedure. The pt usually recovers with very little neurologic deficit with significant improvement in seizure (75% cure rate). Partial frontal, parietal/occipital lobectomy can be performed as well but the result is not as good as temporal lobectomy.
Vagal nerve stimulator, corpus callosotomy, multiple subpial transection, and hemispherectomy are other surgical options for intractable epilepsy if lobectomy is not an option.

IV
Altered Mental Status

In what way is the pt confused?
Most of the time, the pt is unable to provide a history. It is very helpful to obtain history from family members and nursing staff.
It is also important to obtain the pt's baseline mental status.
A reduction in alertness and psychomotor activity is generally seen in acute confusional state which is caused by processes that decreases brain activity such as stroke and infection.
Overactivity, sleeplessness, tremulousness, and prominence of vivid hallucinations are seen in delirium, which is caused by process that increases brain activity such as EtOH withdrawal.

How long has the pt been confused?
Acute confusional state and delirium implies the mental status change is acute and there is a new underlying etiology responsible for the change.
If the pt has been confused chronically over months to years, he or she most likely has dementia.

Is there any new medication started recently?
Review the medication list carefully. Pay attention to possible drug interactions.
Also ask about over-the-counter medication and health supplements used. Many patients do not consider these medications but they can cause altered mental status, especially in elderly.

Are there any constitutional symptoms?
It is best to go through a thorough review of systems with a family member or caretaker. Are there any fever/chills, cough, diarrhea, constipation, weight loss, bright red blood per rectum, dysuria, and sleep disturbances?

Is the pt confused?
Most of the time it is obvious. However, sometimes the confusion is mild and only closest family member will be able to tell. It's helpful to have a family member present when examining pt's mental status.
Check orientation to person, place, and time.
Check attention with digit span forward and backward, spell "world" forward and backward.
Check for recent memory with naming the president, mayor, and details of entry to the hospital.

Perform general physical and neurologic exam
Look for signs of infection: fever, tachypnea, tachycardia, neck stiffness
Look for signs of organ failure: ascites, spider angioma, anasarca, S3, S4
Presence of asterixis is consistent with hepatic encephalopathy
Presence of myoclonus suggests uremia encephalopathy
Perform neurologic exam to assess focality. If there is a focal deficit, then the cause is likely primary CNS. If non-focal, then it's likely metabolic or toxic.

Review basic labs
Electrolytes, glucose, BUN, creatinine, liver function tests, thyroid-stimulating hormone

Altered mental status
Extremely common problem encountered in all hospitals on daily basis.
A useful mnemonic for the possible causes is "VITAMINS"

- Vascular: Stroke and intracranial hemorrhage involving the non-dominant hemisphere or temporal lobes, subarachnoid hemorrhage, venous thrombosis
- Infection: Any infection will cause altered mental status (AMS), especially in elderly pts, urinary tract infection and pneumonia being the most common. Sepsis, endocarditis, fungemia are common in ICU settings. Meningitis and viral encephalitis are the primary CNS infections. Consider opportunistic infections in immunocompromised pts.
- Traumatic: Subdural hematoma, concussion, and contusion
- Autoimmune: Cerebral vasculitis, lupus cerebritis
- Metabolic: Hepatic, kidney, congestive heart failures, electrolyte abnormalities, hyperglycemia and hypoglycemia, hypoxia, hypercapnia, porphyria, endocrinopathies such as hyperthyroidism and hypothyroidism and corticosteroid excess
- Iatrogenic: Medications, drug intoxication/withdrawal: narcotics, barbiturates, sedatives, anticholinergics, antianxieties, antispastics, and corticosteroids
- Neoplasm: Brain tumors, particularly those involving temporal lobes and upper brainstem, carcinomatous meningitis, paraneoplastic syndrome such as limbic encephalitis
- Seizure: Non-convulsive seizures can be difficult to recognize and can certainly cause acute confusional state and bizarre behavior

Establish the cause of AMS and treat the underlying disease
Often there are no clear reasons for the pt's AMS. In these situations, obtain MRI of brain with contrast and perform lumbar puncture. If these are normal, the chance of primary CNS cause of AMS is very low.

Obtain EEG
EEG is an invaluable tool in pts with AMS. It is the only way to diagnose and exclude underlying subclinical seizure.
It can sometimes help to pinpoint the underlying medical illness.

- Triphasic waves are seen in hepatic and uremic encephalopathy.
  - Fast β activity (>14 Hz brain waves) is seen in encephalopathy due to drugs such as benzodiazepine, tricyclic antidepressants, and antipsychotics.

It also has prognostic value in terms of level of brain activity and function.

Protect pt's safety
Ask attendant or family member to stay with pt at all times if possible.
Oral feeding with supervision
Restrain pt if danger to self

Avoid sedatives, narcotics, and other meds that can contribute to AMS

Reassure pt's family
Most confused pts recover if they receive good medical and nursing care.
Depending on the baseline brain reserve, recovery may take days to weeks once the underlying medical disease is under control.

S Is there a known cause of pt's possible brain death? Is it reversible?
One of the prerequisites for diagnosis of brain death is that there has to be a *known, irreversible* CNS catastrophe. This can be fulfilled by clinical or radiologic evidence (e.g., a history of prolonged cardiac arrest or CT evidence of diffuse infarct).

Are there any medical conditions that may confound clinical assessment?
No severe electrolyte, acid-base, endocrine disturbance can be present.

Are there any sedatives or CNS suppressants present?
No benzodiazepines, narcotics, and EtOH should be detected on toxicology screen.

Is there hypothermia?
Core temperature has to be $\geq 32°C$ (90°F).

Are there conditions that might interfere with clinical assessment of brain death?
If any of the following are present then *confirmatory tests* are needed
- Severe facial trauma
- Preexisting pupillary abnormalities
- Toxic level of drugs such as aminoglycoside, tricyclic antidepressants, anticholinergics, anti-epileptic drugs, chemotherapies, neuromuscular blocking agents
- Sleep apnea or severe pulmonary disease resulting in chronic retention of CO_2

Brain death exam
The main goal of neurologic exam in brain death evaluation is to establish absence of BOTH cerebral and brainstem functions.

A. Absence of cerebral function
Suggested by presence of coma
No cerebral motor response to pain in all extremities (nail-bed pressure, sternal rub, and supraorbital pressure)

B. Absence of brainstem function
1. Pupillary reflex (CN2 and CN3)
   - No response to bright light is present
2. Oculocephalic reflex: (CN3, CN6, and CN8)
   - No oculocephalic reflex is present (do not perform on pts on cervical spine precaution)
   - If oculocephalic reflex is absent, perform cold caloric test
     a. Examine both ears with an otoscope to be sure it is s safe to perform the test.
     b. Inject 50 cc of cold water into one ear.
     c. Observe eye movement for 1 min. With intact brainstem, both eyes will slowly deviate toward the side of cold water with fast nystagmus beating to the other side. With brain death, there won't be any movement.
     d. Wait for 5 minutes and repeat step (b) on the other ear.
3. Corneal reflex (CN5 and CN7)
   - Gently touch the corneas with cotton swab and observe for any eye lid movement
4. Gag and cough reflex (CN9, CN10, and CN12)
   - No response after stimulation of the posterior pharynx with endotracheal tube or tongue blade
   - No cough response to bronchial suctioning

Brain Death
Defined as the irreversible loss of function of the brain, including brainstem.
Brain death is a modern medical phenomenon. Brain is required for vital heart and respiratory function. With mechanical ventilation and vasopressors, a brain-dead pt is able to be kept "alive" for prolonged time.
Before proceeding with brain death evaluation, communicate with family and provide option of organ donation.
Once brain death is established, pt is pronounced as clinically dead. There is no hope for any sort of recovery, even to a state of irreversible coma. Artificial life supports must be stopped unless waiting for organ harvesting.

Repeat brain death exam 6 hrs after the first one
Remember to document the etiology and irreversibility of condition.
If on the second exam pt still appears brain dead, perform apnea test:
1. Prerequisites: Core temperature $\geq$ 36.5°C (97°F). Systolic BP $\geq$ 90 mm Hg.
2. Preoxygenate with 100% O_2 for 5 min through the ventilator.
3. Disconnect the ventilator. Continue to deliver 100% O_2 through cannula into the endotracheal tube. Observe for 8 min.
4. Look closely for respiratory movement (chest or abdominal excursions). If pt has spontaneous breathing then apnea test is negative and pt is not brain dead.
5. If systolic BP drops below 90 mm Hg or pt goes into cardiac arrhythmia, reconnect ventilator and stop the test. Perform confirmatory test.
6. Draw ABG at the end of 8 min. Reconnect ventilator.
7. If PCO_2 is $\geq$ 60 mm Hg or $\geq$ 20 mm Hg above baseline, then the apnea test is positive (i.e., pt is brain dead). If not then the result is indeterminate, and an additional confirmatory test can be considered.
8. Document the results in the chart. Notify primary physician.

Consider confirmatory tests
A confirmatory test should be obtained when a complete standard brain death evaluation is not feasible.
Any of the following is an acceptable confirmatory test listed in the order of the most sensitive test first.
1. Conventional angiography
    - No intracerebral filling at the level of the carotid bifurcation or circle of Willis.
2. EEG (the most commonly used confirmatory test)
    - No electrical activity during at least 30 minutes of brain death protocol recording.
3. Transcranial Doppler ultrasonography
    - Absence of diastolic flow in intracerebral vessels.
4. Technetium-99m hexamethylpropyleneamineoxime brain scan
    - No uptake of isotope in brain parenchyma ("hollow skull phenomenon").
5. Somatosensory-evoked potentials
    - Absence of bilateral N20-P22 (cerebral) response with median nerve stimulation.

Wernicke-Korsakoff Syndrome

S — **Does the pt have symptoms of Wernicke encephalopathy?**
Most of the time pts with Wernicke encephalopathy are brought in by family or police for mental status change. A history of confusion, apathy, inattention, amnesia, and confabulation is often given by the family or police report.
Sometimes, pts may voluntarily complain of the following symptoms:
- Visual disturbances: Double vision and strabismus
- Gait abnormalities: Unsteady gait, frequent falls

O — **Assess mental status**
Most common presentation is global confusional state. Pt is disoriented, inattentive, and unaware of the surroundings.
In severe cases, pts may be in stupor or coma.
Often pt will present with EtOH withdrawal characterized by restless, agitation, hallucination.

Assess for evidence of Korsakoff psychosis
Hallmarks of Korsakoff psychosis are memory disturbance and confabulation.
The memory disturbance is characterized by both retrograde and anterograde amnesia. To assess retrograde amnesia, ask questions such as the pt's birthday, or to name the president. To assess for anterograde amnesia, ask the pt to perform a 1-minute recall on three objects.
Confabulation is the filling-in of gaps in memory to make a coherent story. Fact and fantasy become inextricably intermingled. For example, when asked what the pt did the previous night, he/she might say "I went to a movie last night," when indeed the pt was in the hospital. The pt is unaware the answer given is incorrect.

Assess extraocular movements
Nystagmus is the most common ocular sign and can be present in both horizontal and vertical gaze.
Often bilateral lateral rectus weakness is observed. Both eyes are not able to abduct. An internal strabismus may be seen.
In severe cases, pt may have ophthalmoplegia in which both eyes have restricted conjugated gazes in all directions.
Rarely the pupils will be affected and become miotic and nonreactive to light.

Assess gait and ataxia
Observe for wide-based gait, which is a sign of unsteadiness.
If pt is able to walk well, check for tandem walk to bring out subtle ataxia.
If pt is not able to get out of bed, then do heel-shin test.

Assess for evidence of peripheral neuropathy
Peripheral neuropathy is very common in Wernicke encephalopathy pts. If pt has peripheral neuropathy, recovery of gait function will be more difficult.
Peripheral neuropathy is most evident in the distal lower extremities. The most sensitive modality to test is vibratory sense. Use a 256-Hz tuning fork and compare between distal and proximal area of lower legs.
Also ask pt to perform Romberg test (standing with eyes closed and feet together). It tests lower extremity proprioception.

Wernicke-Korsakoff syndrome
Incidence of Wernicke-Korsakoff affects approximately 2% of the general population.
Onset is usually between 30 and 70 years of age, with males affected slightly more than females.
It carries a mortality rate of 10% to 20%. Prompt diagnosis and treatment is crucial.
The classic triad of Wernicke disease is *ophthalmoplegia, ataxia,* and *altered mental status*. If left untreated, Korsakoff syndrome will develop, which is characterized by amnesia and confabulation.

The syndrome is caused by deficiency of dietary thiamine, which is a B vitamin that is required for glucose utilization. Mammillary bodies, thalamus, hypothalamus, midbrain, and cerebellum are affected more than other areas of brain. Microscopically, intense vascular proliferation, dilation, and leakage are seen along with gliosis and macrophage infiltration. Neurons are spared at this time.

If treatment is not instituted in a timely fashion neuronal cell death occurs and the damage is irreversible.

The causes of Wernicke-Korsakoff syndrome include:
1. Chronic alcoholism (most common)
2. Malnutrition such as anorexia nervosa, hyperemesis gravidarum, and GI diseases
3. Iatrogenic causes such as intravenous hyperalimentation (e.g., huge carbohydrate load after prolonged starving) and chronic hemodialysis
4. Systemic disease such as AIDS, malignancy, tuberculosis

Start IV thiamine
Because prompt treatment will stop the progress of the disease and reverse some of the symptoms before permanent structural damage occurs, it is imperative to start treatment on all cases suspected of Wernicke.

Give thiamine 100 mg IV bolus for one dose followed by daily doses of 50–100 mg IV/IM/PO until pt is able to resume regular diet. After that a daily multivitamin tablet should be sufficient.

Chronic alcoholics often are deficient in magnesium and potassium as well. The Mg and K levels should be checked and replaced as needed.

Do not give IV fluid containing glucose with thiamine because glucose may exhaust pt's already low thiamine reserve and precipitate full blown Wernicke encephalopathy.

Ocular signs will resolve within days after infusion of thiamine. Failure to do so should raise possibility of another diagnosis.

Korsakoff amnesic psychotic state has poorer prognosis. Only 20% will have resolution of symptoms and recovery takes weeks to months.

Initiate physical therapy for gait training
Ataxia will resolve in approximately 40% of pts. Other pts will have permanent gait difficulties and require physical therapy for gait training. Prescribe walkers or canes if needed.

Attempt to refer pt to Alcoholic Anonymous or other self-help program
Abstinence from alcohol is needed to achieve optimal recovery.
Physician should attempt to break the cycle of pt drinking and getting sick.
It is the most important part of treatment but is often overlooked.

V
CNS Infectious Disease

Bacterial Meningitis

S **Does the pt have the classic symptoms and signs of bacterial meningitis?**
Severe headache, fever, and neck stiffness

What is the age of the pt and the most likely organism?
Neonate: *E. coli*, Group B streptococcus
Children: *H. influenzae*, pneumococcus, meningococcus
Adolescent: pneumococcus, meningococcus
Adult: pneumococcus, meningococcus, *H. influenza*, *Listeria*, and staphylococcus

What is the clinical setting and the most likely organism?
Community-acquired: pneumococcus, *H. influenza*, meningococcus
Nosocomial: Gram-negative bacilli and staphylococcus
Post-surgical: staphylococcus

Any underlying medical illness putting pt susceptible to certain organism?
Splenectomized, sickle cell, and chronic alcoholic pts are more susceptible to pneumococcus.
Immunocompromised pts with HIV, myeloproliferative disorders, or chemotherapy are likely to have *Enterobacteriaceae*, *Listeria*, *A. calcoaceticus*, and *Pseudomonas*.

Are there symptoms of concomitant infection in other parts of body?
Ask about cough, ear pain, and sinus pain for pneumonia, otitis, and sinusitis, respectively

Perform quick physical and neurologic exam
Bacterial meningitis is a medical emergency with high morbidity and mortality. Make the diagnosis and start appropriate treatment quickly.
Check vital signs
Neck stiffness
Look for papilledema for elevated intracranial pressure (ICP)
Brudzinski (involuntary flexion at the hip and knee in response to passive flexion of the neck)
Kernig sign (inability to completely extend the legs with hips flexed)
Auscultate lung, examine tympanic membranes and oropharynx
Look for signs of petechial or purpuric rash in meningococcal septicemia

Perform lumbar puncture
If on exam there is focal findings or signs of increased ICP, then a head CT should be done before lumbar puncture. However, in the majority of cases, this is not necessary and should not delay the diagnosis and treatment.
Obtain opening pressure
- A normal opening pressure (<180 mm H_2O) argues against bacterial meningitis or raises the possibility that the spinal subarachnoid space is blocked by pockets of exudate.
- Pressures over 400 mm H_2O suggest the presence of brain swelling and the potential for herniation. Consult neurosurgery for ventriculostomy.

Pleocytosis is diagnostic of bacterial meningitis.
- Cell count in cerebrospinal fluid (CSF) is usually 250 to approximately 10,000/mm^3 with >85% neutrophils.
- If cell count >50,000/mm^3, the likely diagnosis is a ruptured brain abscess into ventricle.

Protein content is high, in ranges of 100 to 500 mg/dL.
Glucose is low, less than 40 mg/dL or less than 40% of serum glucose value.
Sent for Gram stain and culture, results of which are positive in 70% to 90% of cases.

Bacterial Meningitis
Pneumococcus, meningococcus, and *H. influenza* account for > 75% of all cases of bacterial meningitis.
Cases occur worldwide and mainly during fall, winter, and spring.
Pyogenic infection reaches the CNS either by hematogenous spread or by extension from cranial structures (ears, paranasal sinuses).
After the bacteria reach the subarachnoid space, they spread through the entire CSF space around the brain, spinal cord, and optic nerves.
The meningeal venules and capillaries respond by increase permeability, allowing migration of neutrophils and exudation of proteins into the pia and subarachnoid space.
The neutrophils then phagocytize bacteria and release cytokines recruiting lymphocytes, plasma cells, macrophages, and fibroblasts.

Complications
Intense inflammation surrounding the blood vessels causes *thrombosis*, which is more common in veins than in arteries.
There may be *focal infarcts* and necrosis in brain tissues surrounding these vessels, causing nerve damage. As a result, *neurologic deficits* and *seizures* may develop.
Thick inflammatory exudates in the CSF space may obstruct the foramina of Magendie and Luschka or other subarachnoid tight spaces, causing acute *obstructive hydrocephalus*.
In later stages, fibrous subarachnoid adhesions interfere with CSF absorption and causes *non-obstructive hydrocephalus*.

Start empiric antibiotics
Antibiotics should be started while awaiting the results of Gram stain/culture and should be changed later in accordance with the culture result.
- 0 to 4 wks   cefotaxime + ampicillin
- 4 to 12 wks 3rd gen. cephalosporin + ampicillin
- 3 months to 50 y/o 3rd gen. cephalosporin + vancomycin
- > 50 y/o 3rd gen. cephalosporin + vancomycin + ampicillin
- Immunocompromised   Vancomycin + ampicillin + ceftazidime
- Basilar skill fracture 3rd gen. cephalosporin + vancomycin
- Neurosurgery, shunts   vancomycin + ceftazidime

Consider steroids
Steroids reduce the incidence of sensorineural deafness and other neurologic sequelae associated with bacterial meningitis, especially in children.
It is generally recommended to start steroids in cases of severe bacterial meningitis. Start dexamethasone 0.15 mg/kg Q 6 hrs for 4 days. Make sure to write an order to check fingerstick QAC and QHS; give GI prophylaxis and potassium supplement.

Does the pt have these symptoms of encephalitis?
Headache and fever are the most common symptoms.
Other symptoms include seizures, confusion, stupor, and coma.

Is there a preexisting history of oral or genital herpes?
In adults, herpes simplex virus (HSV) encephalitis is almost always due to HSV-1, which is also the cause of common herpetic lesions of the oral mucosa.
In neonate, HSV encephalitis is usually due to HSV-2 in relation to maternal genital herpetic infection.

Is there a history of insect or mosquito bite?
Many arthropod-borne viruses (arbovirus) cause encephalitis. Their life cycle requires viremic hosts (horse or bird). Infection occurs after the mosquito injects virus into human.
Rabies causes encephalitis and sometimes Guillain-Barré–like flaccid paralysis. It is caused by bites from animals such as wild dogs, skunks, and bats.

What is the season and location?
HSV encephalitis is by far the most common sporadic cause of encephalitis and has no seasonal or geographic predilections.
Epidemic viral encephalitis is principally caused by arboviruses. Many have characteristic geographic and seasonal incidence. They usually occur in outbreaks. So ask about travel history and any other people ill in the neighborhood.
- Eastern equine virus: mainly on East Coast; least common but most lethal
- Western equine virus: west of Mississippi; quite common but benign
- St. Louis virus: Mississippi River during summer and fall; most common
- Venezuelan equine virus: Florida and southwestern states
- California and La Crosse virus: northern Midwest and northeastern states
- West Nile virus: mainly during summer season, seen across the U.S.

 Perform a general physical and neurologic exam
Pt usually has low grade fever.
Meningeal signs such as photophobia and stiff neck may be present.
Mental status is often abnormal, ranging from delirium and bizarre behavior to stupor and coma.
Focal signs such as aphasia, hemiparesis.
Pupillary change and coma may be from temporal lobe edema/herniation or virus affecting upper brainstem.

Perform MRI of brain with/without contrast
Except for HSV encephalitis, MRI is often not very helpful and is ordered mainly to rule out other causes.
The classic finding for HSV encephalitis is bilateral temporal lobe increase signal on T2 sequence with enhancement on T1 after contrast sequence.

Perform lumbar puncture
It is the most important test to establish the diagnosis.
For HSV encephalitis, opening pressure is often mildly elevated. WBC is elevated (range 10 to 500 cells/mm^3) with predominantly lymphocytes. RBC can range from 0 to thousands with xanthochromia. Protein is increased and glucose may be slightly decreased.
Send cerebrospinal fluid HSV polymerase chain reaction (PCR) study, which has sensitivity of approximately 98%. Antiviral treatment does not appear to affect the test. So do not delay treatment waiting for lumbar puncture.

Obtain EEG

Classic HSV finding is PLEDS (periodic lateralizing epileptic discharges), which are high voltage sharp waves and slow-wave complexes at two- to three-per-second intervals seen in the temporal lobes.

EEG is also useful in ruling out ongoing subclinical status epilepticus, which is common in pts with encephalitis.

Herpes and other viral encephalitides

Encephalitis is the infection of brain parenchyma whereas meningitis is infection of meninges. Viral meningitis is also called aseptic meningitis and is usually self-limited.

In the U.S., there are approximately 20,000 cases of acute viral encephalitis reported every year. Mortality is approximately 20% and morbidity is approximately another 20%.

There is a large number of viruses capable of causing encephalitis; however, only a few occur with sufficient frequency to have diagnostic importance.

HSV is by far the most common sporadic cause of encephalitis, accounting for approximately 20% of all viral encephalitis cases in U.S.

The age distribution is biphasic, between 5 and 30 years of age and in those older than 50.

It has a high mortality rate of 70% if left untreated and high morbidity. Approximately 40% of survivors are left with serious neurologic deficits.

HSV-1 remains dormant in trigeminal ganglion after initial infection. With reactivation, it spread along fibers that innervate the leptomeninges of the anterior and middle fossa. Therefore the lesions are localized to temporal lobes and medial-orbital parts of the frontal lobes.

It causes a *hemorrhagic* necrosis in the temporal lobes (↑ CSF RBC).

Intranuclear eosinophilic inclusion bodies (Cowdry A) are seen on biopsy specimen.

Stabilize pt

Often pt with HSV encephalitis presents with obtundation and coma. Intubate pt for airway protection.

If pupillary change and coma are seen, rule out herniation by imaging and follow appropriate measures. They can also be present from the virus infecting upper brainstem, which carries grave prognosis.

Start pt on IV anticonvulsants if there is evidence of clinical or subclinical seizure on EEG.

Start antiviral medication

Acyclovir 30 mg/kg IV QD for 14 days.

Acyclovir should be started in all suspected cases of encephalitis. It does not seem to alter CSF PCR results. It can be started before performing lumbar puncture and discontinued once HSV is ruled out.

Main side effects include local vein irritation, mild elevation of liver function tests, and transient impairment of renal function. Overall, it is a very well-tolerated medication and side effects are rarely seen.

If treatment is started within 4 days of onset of illness in conscious pts, survival is > 90%.

If the mental status is poor, so is the outcome.

Neurosyphilis

S **Does the pt have symptoms of neurosyphilis?**
Syphilis is known as the "great masquerader." It can mimic any disease with a variety of presentations.
Pts with neurosyphilis can present with any one of the following syndromes:
- Asymptomatic syphilis (0 to 1 year after initial inoculation).
    - Pt is asymptomatic. Diagnosis is purely incidental.
- Meningeal syphilis (0 to 2 years after initial inoculation).
    - Headache, stiff neck, cranial nerve palsies, seizure, mental confusion.
- Meningovascular syphilis (6 to 7 years after initial inoculation).
    - Ischemic stroke due to invasion of arteries.
- Paretic neurosyphilis (15 to 20 years after initial inoculation).
    - Memory loss, impairment of reasoning, dementia, dysarthria, tremor, seizure.
- Tabes dorsalis (15 to 20 years after initial inoculation).
    - Lancinating pains in extremities, ataxia, urinary incontinence, diplopia.
- Syphilitic optic atrophy (15 to 20 years after initial inoculation).
    - Blurry vision, blindness in one or both eyes.

Does the pt have risk factors for syphilis?
Syphilis is a sexually transmitted disease. Ask for sexual history, especially unprotected sex.

 Perform a general and neurologic physical exam
Examine the skin and genital for rash or chancre.
Check for generalized lymphadenopathy.

Look for Argyll Robertson pupil
- The pupils fail to react to light, although they do constrict on accommodation (light near dissociation).
- Sign of late stage neurosyphilis, seen in tabes dorsalis.

Look for signs of stroke (e.g., hemiparesis, hemisensory loss)
Perform a detailed sensory exam in both feet. In tabes dorsalis, pt will have decreased vibratory and proprioceptive sensory loss in both feet. Romberg will be positive. Ankle reflexes are diminished or absent.

Screen pts with serum rapid plasma reagin (RPR) or Venereal Disease Research Laboratories (VDRL) testing
Because syphilis can present like every other neurologic disease and is highly treatable, it should be included in the differential diagnosis of all neurology pts.
There are two types of antibodies used to detect syphilis
1. Nonspecific or nontreponemal antibodies (high sensitivity)
    a. RPR
    b. VDRL
2. Specific treponemal antibodies (high specificity)
    a. Fluorescent treponemal antibody absorption (FTA-ABS)
    b. Microhemagglutination assay for *Treponema pallidum* (MHA-TP)

RPR and VDRL are good screening tests for syphilis. One or the other should be ordered for all pts with neurologic symptoms.
Serum RPR and VDRL test results can be falsely positive after immunization, in acute viral infection, or during pregnancy.
Serum RPR and VDRL test results can also be falsely negative in some pts with late syphilis and neurosyphilis.
To confirm syphilis, order FTA-ABS or MHA-TP.

Perform lumbar puncture
CSF is required to diagnose neurosyphilis
CSF abnormalities in neurosyphilis include:
1. Pleocytosis: cell count is around 100/mm^3, and consists predominantly of lymphocytes
2. Increased protein: from 40–200 mg/dL
3. Increase in IgG
4. Positive serologic test result (VDRL): is diagnostic of neurosyphilis

Neurosyphilis
Syphilis is caused by *T. pallidum*, a slender and spiral bacterium.

It can only survive briefly outside the body, so transmission almost always requires direct contact with the infected lesion. It enters the body through minute abrasions on skin or mucous membrane.

The treponeme usually invades the CNS within 3 to 8 months of inoculation. In small minority of pts with syphilis, the organism never invades the CNS and neurosyphilis does not occur.

Once the treponeme enters the CNS, it causes meningitis. Usually the meningitis is asymptomatic and can be discovered only by lumbar puncture. Some pts do get full-blown meningitis with fever, headache, seizure, and cranial nerve palsies.

From a clinical point of view, asymptomatic neurosyphilis stage is the most important form of neurosyphilis. If asymptomatic neurosyphilis is caught and treated, late forms of neurosyphilis will not develop.

Because asymptomatic neurosyphilis can only be detected by lumbar puncture, it is recommended that all pts with syphilis found incidentally get lumbar puncture.

Treat with antibiotics
Once the diagnosis of neurosyphilis is made, treat pt with either
    Penicillin G 4 million units IV Q 4 hrs for 14 days
        Or
    Erythromycin 500 mg PO Q 6 hrs for 30 days AND
    Tetracycline 500 mg PO Q 6 hrs for 30 days

Follow-up
Have pt follow-up 3 months after treatment to see if symptoms improve.
Repeat lumbar puncture 6 months after treatment.
If symptoms resolve and CSF normalizes (normal cell count/protein with negative or weakly positive VDRL), then no further treatment is needed.
If CSF is still abnormal, then start another course of antibiotic treatment.
This process should be repeated every 3 and 6 months until the CSF profile normalizes.

Neurocysticercosis — CNS Infectious Disease

S
Has the pt had a seizure or other focal neurologic complaint?
The most common presentation of neurocysticercosis is focal seizure. The seizure may or may not secondarily generalize so the pt may or may not lose consciousness.
Headache, nausea, and vomiting are common also if there is ↑ intracranial pressure (ICP).
Less often pt may present with hemiparesis or numbness.

What is the pt's ethnicity?
Cysticercosis is very prevalent in Central and South America. It is present in parts of Africa, Asia, and Middle East as well.
If pt is Hispanic and has seizures, the diagnosis is cysticercosis until proven otherwise. In southern and western U.S., cysticercosis is very common due to Hispanic immigration.

Is there travel history and contact with people from endemic areas?
Be sure to ask about travel history to endemic areas. The infection can precede symptoms by as long as 5 years.
Because cysticercosis is transmitted fecal-orally, ask about contacts with visitors from endemic areas.

O
Perform a general physical and neurologic exam
Most pts with neurocysticercosis have a normal exam.
Transient hemiparesis may be present immediately after convulsion due to the postictal hypoactivity at the seizure focus (Todd's paralysis).
If the cyst is intraventricular or in the subarachnoid space causing obstruction, pt may exhibit signs of increased intracranial pressure.

Obtain head CT with contrast
The presence of punctate calcification in brain is diagnostic of cysticercosis if clinical picture fits.
The calcifications are dead neurocysticercosis. Live cysts may not be seen on CT scan.

Consider MRI of brain with contrast
MRI may or may not be diagnostic. Sometimes the scolex of the parasite can be seen and is diagnostic of neurocysticercosis.

Consider lumbar puncture
If other infectious etiology is suspected.
In approximately 50% of cases, lymphocytic pleocytosis can be detected along with low glucose, increased protein, and elevated opening pressure.
Presence of eosinophils in CSF strongly support the diagnosis of cysticercosis.

Consider checking cysticercosis titer
Enzyme-linked immunotransfer blot (EITB) or enzyme-linked immunosorbent assay (ELISA) can be sent.
These test results can show whether pt has been exposed to cysticercosis. They may not be helpful if pt comes from endemic area because majority of population has been exposed.

Test stool for ova and parasite
If positive result, pt should be treated to prevent further spread of disease.

Neurocysticercosis
Caused by the pork tapeworm *Taenia solium*.
The life cycle of *T. solium*:
- Humans with infected tapeworm in their intestine shed eggs or gravid proglottids (which carry about 50,000 eggs each) in feces and passed into the environment.
- Pigs or human eat food contaminated with feces. The eggs hatch into oncospheres in the intestine.
- The oncospheres invade the intestinal wall and migrate to CNS (brain, CSF space, and spinal cord), striated muscle, eyes, and other tissues, where they develop into cysticerci. The cysticerci in the brain cause neurocysticercosis.
- Human eats undercooked pork containing cysticerci. Cysts evaginate and attach to the small intestine and develop into adult tapeworms.
- The adult tapeworms shed eggs and gravid proglottids, which are released with human feces.

Note that eating undercooked pork with cysticerci will only produce tapeworm infection. Neurocysticercosis will only develop if the human ingests eggs through fecal oral contamination.

Neurocysticercosis is divided into four stages:
- Vesicular stage: The cysticerci is alive and with minimal inflammation. This stage can last 2 to 6 years and pt is usually asymptomatic.
- Colloid stage: The worm inside the cyst dies and triggers host immune cells to enter the cyst fluid. Intense inflammation surrounding the cyst causes severe symptoms.
- Granular-nodular stage: The cyst cavity collapses and fibrosis occurs.
- Calcified stage: The dead worm decays into a tiny calcified mass and remains in the brain permanently.

Treat acute symptoms first
Start an anti-epileptic medication if pt has seizure.
If pt has signs of ↑ ICP, treat obstructive hydrocephalus first.

Decide whether or not to treat the neurocysticercosis
There is no standard guideline regarding treatment of neurocysticercosis.
Argument against treating neurocysticercosis:
- All cysts eventually die by themselves.
- Treatment with antihelmetics carries risks (bursting of the cysts causes intense inflammation).

Argument for treating neurocysticercosis:
- Treatment with antihelmetics seems to decrease chance of developing recurrent seizure.
- Treatment will break the life-cycle of the parasite if pt carries adult tapeworm. So the pt will not be able to self-inoculate with eggs and develop more neurocysticercosis.

Treating neurocysticercosis
Admit pt to hospital for the first 5 to 7 days of treatment.
Start praziquantel 50 mg/kg PO QD for 15 days or albendazole 5 mg/kg PO TID for 15 days.
Concomitantly administer prednisone or dexamethasone to minimize inflammation.

Educate pt
Emphasize the importance of hand-washing and cooking pork thoroughly.

S **Does the pt have prodrome symptoms?**
Approximately one third of pts with Creutzfeldt-Jakob disease (CJD) complain of fatigue, depression, weight loss, poor appetite, and insomnia several weeks before onset of illness.

Are there mental status or personality changes?
In early stage of disease, pts present with changes in behavior, emotional response, and intellectual function. There may be hallucination, delusion, and agitation as well. The mental deterioration progresses rapidly over weeks to dementia and muteness.

What other neurologic symptoms does the pt have?
Very frequently pt will complain of ataxia and visual disturbances.
Headache, vertigo, sensory symptoms, and speech change in form of dysarthria are common as well.

What is the time course of the symptoms?
Symptoms of CJD start insidiously and progress rapidly over the course of several weeks. If symptoms develop over many months to years, consider a different diagnosis of dementia.

Is there a family history of CJD or similar dementing illness?
Approximately 10% of CJD cases are familial. The mutation is in the gene that encodes the prion protein (PrP) in the short arm of chromosome 20.

Are there risk factors for getting CJD?
The spread of CJD is mainly iatrogenic. Known risk factors include:
- History of corneal or dural graft transplantation.
- History of receiving human gonadotropic or growth hormone prepared from pooled cadaveric pituitary glands.
- History of intracranial electrode placement or contact with infected neurosurgical instruments. At least one neurosurgeon is known to have acquired CJD.

Assess mental status
Most pts present with dementia, followed by muted state, and then progress to stupor and coma at end stage.
The startle response is strikingly exaggerated in CJD. Clap hands loudly and pt will be startled out of proportion.

Assess cerebellar function
Look for nystagmus. Vertical nystagmus is a sign of cerebellar dysfunction.
Finger-nose-finger test may demonstrate dysmetria. Gait is ataxic and impaired.

Look for myoclonus
Myoclonus is a sudden, involuntary jerking of a muscle or group of muscles.
Myoclonus usually develops in CJD pts after dementia started. It is seen in > 80% of pts with CJD.
The myoclonic jerks may be spontaneous and can be evoked by sensory or tactile stimuli (startle myoclonus).

Look for pyramidal tract signs
They are present in > 50% of pts with CJD. Signs include spasticity, hyperreflexia, positive Babinski sign.

Perform lumbar puncture
CJD does not evoke immune or inflammatory response. CSF profile is normal. Protein is normal in most cases but can be slightly elevated.

CSF protein 14-3-3 is the diagnostic test for CJD and has sensitivity of 96% and specificity of 99%.

CSF should also be sent for Venereal Disease Research Laboratories testing and measles titer to rule out neurosyphilis and subacute sclerosing panencephalitis (SSPE).

Order EEG

Classic EEG finding in CJD is high-voltage slow (1 to 2 Hz) and sharp-wave complexes on an increasingly slow and low-voltage background.

Consider brain MRI

Brain MRI is obtained to exclude other treatable causes. It may show nonspecific ↑ signal on bilateral basal ganglia in approximately 80% of pts.

Creutzfeldt-Jakob disease

CJD is a rare disease, occurring in approximately 2 per million people but has received considerable media attention due to British outbreak of "mad cow disease."

It is one of the *transmissible spongiform encephalopathies*, which includes CJD, Kuru, Gerstmann-Sträussler-Scheinker, and fatal familial insomnia, all of which are caused by prions, which are infectious proteins.

A prion is a normal sialoglycoprotein presented on host cell membranes. The prion protein causing the diseases is an isoform of the normal prion protein.

The abnormal protein has a large β-sheet content compare to normal protein, which has predominant α-helical structure.

The normal native prion protein is susceptible to undergo this conformation change (from α-helix or β-sheet) when in contact with the abnormal protein. This is responsible for the propagation of the altered protein in brain tissue.

The abnormal prion protein is protease resistant, thus accumulates in neural cells, leading to vacuolization and cell death. Under the microscope, the brain tissue appears like a sponge; hence, the name spongiform encephalopathy.

Mad cow disease (bovine spongiform encephalopathy) is a prion disease affecting cows. When humans eat infected cow, the person may develop what is now called "new variant CJD." These pts are younger, with prominent early psychiatric and behavior manifestations compared to traditional CJD. Sensory complaints are more common.

The differential diagnosis of CJD (*dementia* + *myoclonus* + *cerebellar signs*) includes lithium intoxication, Hashimoto encephalopathy, Whipple disease, carcinomatous meningitis, SSPE, cerebellar lipidosis.

Provide supportive care

There is no specific treatment for CJD. Most die within 1 year from onset.

Take special precautions in medical care

The exact mode of transmission of prion disease is still not certain. Extra precautions should be taken.

Prion is resistant to treatments that inactivate nucleic acids and viruses (boiling, alcohol, formaldehyde, UV radiation, proteases, and nucleases). However, prions are inactivated by treatments that disrupt proteins (autoclaving, phenol, detergents, and extremes of pH).

Needles, glassware, electrodes, and surgical equipments that come in contact with the pt should be appropriately disinfected or incinerated.

These pts should never be considered as donors for organ transplant.

S **Does the pt recall a tick bite in the previous year?**
The late neurologic symptoms of Lyme disease can occur up to a year after the initial tick bite. However the bite is sometimes innocuous, and 30% of pts with Lyme disease do not recall such an event.

Was there skin rash and flu-like illness?
Erythema migrans develops around the site of bite within 30 days. The rash resolves in 2 to 3 weeks without treatment.
Constitutional symptoms such as fever, myalgia, and arthralgia are common.
Approximately one third of pts will have no further symptoms. Late symptoms of Lyme disease will develop in two thirds of pts.

Does the pt have the acute symptoms of Lyme disease?
A few weeks after the initial disseminated disease, acute neuroborreliosis occurs in approximately 15% of untreated pts.
Symptoms include aseptic meningitis/encephalitis (headache, fever, nausea, vomiting), facial nerve palsy (can be uni-or bilateral facial weakness), optic neuritis (blurry vision), radiculitis (weakness/numbness over particular nerve root), mononeuritis multiplex (wrist drop, foot drop), and myelitis (para-or quadriparesis).
Treatment at this point will cure the disease and reverse the symptoms. Without treatment, the symptoms will eventually resolve in weeks to months.

Does the pt have the late symptoms of Lyme disease?
In approximately 5% of untreated pts, there will be a chronic form of Lyme disease.
Symptoms include chronic peripheral neuropathy (pain, numbness, and weakness in both radicular and non-radicular pattern), myelopathy (para- or quadriparesis), and encephalopathy (confusion, cognitive decline).

Are there other symptoms that might suggest Lyme disease?
Weeks and months after the initial infection, cardiac and joint involvement will occur. Symptoms include joint pain and swelling, chest pain, arrhythmia, and pericarditis.

O **Assess vital signs**
Look for cardiac arrhythmia.
Fever may be present during meningitis phase.

Perform general exam
Examine the skin for erythema migrans (a solitary, expanding, ring-like erythematous lesion), which will probably have disappeared by the time a neurologist is involved.
Look for joint tenderness and swelling.
Auscultate the heart for pericarditis rub and look for signs of cardiac failure.
Palpate for lymphadenopathy.
Check abdomen for hepatosplenomegaly.

Perform complete neurologic exam
Because Lyme disease can strike anywhere in the neurologic axis, a detailed and complete exam is warranted. Pay extra attention to the areas of complaint.

Send laboratory studies
Serum IgG and IgM antibodies to *B. burgdorferi*. If initial ELISA test results are positive, confirmatory Western blot should be performed.
If both IgM and IgG are positive, it strongly supports recent infection. If only IgG is positive, it only means that pt has been exposed to the organism.
If pt has joint swelling, the joint should be tapped and synovial fluid send for culture and polymerase chain reaction test. It has high sensitivity.

Consider lumbar puncture

CSF usually shows lymphocytosis with elevated proteins. Glucose is normal.
IgM and IgG antibodies to *B. burgdorferi* should be sent. Index of CSF to serum antibody ratio should be obtained. It is possible to have intrathecal antibody without serum titer being positive.

Lyme disease

There are approximately 13,000 reported cases annually, mostly in northeastern and north central states. Most infections are acquired from May to July.

The disease is caused by *B. burgdorferi*, a spirochete, and the body's immune response to the infection. It is transmitted through *Ixodes* (deer tick) bite.

B. burgdorferi requires either field mouse or white-tailed deer as its host. When a tick bites and feeds on an infected host, the bacteria enters the tick. When the tick bites a human, the bacteria are transmitted and infection starts.

The tick must be attached to the human for 2 to 3 days to pass on the infection. The number of bacteria in a tick is small but will start to multiply in tick once it bites and starts feeding. The bacteria then migrate to the salivary gland and are injected into the human.

Once the bacteria enter a human, one of three events can happen:
- The pt's immune system kills the bacteria and no symptom occurs.
- *B. burgdorferi* overcomes the human immune system and disseminates through the body causing acute disease.
- *B. burgdorferi* induces abnormal immune response (auto-antibody formation) that leads to many later disease manifestations including arthritis, encephalopathy, and cardiomyositis.

Treat with antibiotics

If the disease is in early state (erythema migrans), treatment with doxycycline 100 mg PO QID or amoxicillin 1000 mg PO TID is adequate.

By the time a neurologist is involved, the disease is usually in a late stage. Treat with third-generation cephalosporin IV for 4 weeks.

Either ceftriaxone 2 g IV QD or cefotaxime 2 g IV Q 8 hrs for 28 days is adequate.

Prognosis

The acute neurologic symptoms (meningitis, facial palsy) usually resolve within weeks. The chronic symptoms (encephalopathy, peripheral neuropathy) may or may not improve. Improvement may take months.

CNS Infectious Disease

S **Does the pt have symptoms of an opportunistic CNS infection?**
Opportunistic organisms can infect the CNS in a variety of ways: meningitis, encephalitis, abscess, and angioinvasion.
The symptoms of meningitis (headache, fever, neck stiffness) due to opportunistic infections are similar to those caused by other organisms, but are milder and develop slower, usually over 1 to 2 weeks.
Seizures, confusion, coma, and focal neurologic complaints such as double vision, dysarthria, hemiparesis, and hemisensory loss.

Does the pt have risk factors for an immunocompromised state?
HIV, chemotherapy, diabetes, alcoholism, congenital immunodeficiency.

O **Perform general physical and neurologic exam**
Vital signs: fever, tachycardia, and tachypnea.
Clues of HIV infection with generalized lymphadenopathy and skin lesions.
Check for nuchal rigidity, Kernig and Brudzinski signs.
Stupor and coma suggest lesions affecting bilateral hemispheres or reticular activating system in brainstem. These may also be signs of pending herniation from hydrocephalus.
Check fundi for papilledema as sign of increased intracranial pressure (ICP).
Cranial nerve signs (ocular palsies, facial weakness/numbness, deafness) suggest basilar meningitis.
Focal neurologic signs such as aphasia, visual field cuts, ataxia, hemiparesis, and hemisensory loss indicate mass lesion or stroke as result of infection.

Obtain brain imaging
MRI with contrast is required but CT scan can be obtained initially to rule out processes requiring immediate attention (e.g., herniation, bleeding).

The MRI findings for the most common opportunistic infection in brain are:
- Multiple nodular or ring-enhancing lesions: toxoplasmosis
- Multiple large area non-enhancing white matter lesions — progressive multifocal leukoencephalitis (PML)
- Enhancing basal meninges (surrounding brainstem and base of hemispheres) with or without hydrocephalus: TB, cryptococcal, and other fungal meningitis

Obtain CSF sample
Perform lumbar puncture if there is no large mass with mass effect and no obstructive hydrocephalus. If neurosurgical intervention is needed for hydrocephalus and herniation, CSF can be obtained during shunt placement.
Lymphocytic and monocytic pleocytosis with elevated protein and subnormal glucose is seen most commonly with TB and fungal infections.
Polymorphonuclear pleocytosis can be seen in early TB or fungal infection.
Normal CSF profile is seen in PML.
CSF should be sent for bacterial and fungal stain and culture. Latex agglutination test for cryptococcus, TB polymerase chain reaction (PCR), cytology, JC virus titer (for PML) can be sent in suspected cases.

Check for evidence of systemic TB, fungal infection, and HIV
Obtain CXR to look for evidence of TB or other fungal infections such as aspergillosis, coccidioidomycosis, and histoplasmosis.
Place PPD with controls
Send HIV test

CNS Infectious Disease — Opportunistic Infections

Toxoplasmosis

Is caused by the ubiquitous protozoal parasite *Toxoplasma gondii*, an obligate intracellular organism identified by Wright- or Giemsa stain.

Infection can be acquired or congenital. Congenital infection is caused by parasitemia of mother during pregnancy. Acquired infection is by eating raw/undercooked beef, mutton, and contact with cat feces.

The organism causes multiple foci of necrotizing encephalitis with surrounding edema. Antibody test is not useful because most of people are exposed to it. Diagnosis is usually clinical and radiological.

TB Meningitis

Is caused by *Mycobacterium tuberculosis*, which enters through inhalation. The organism then reaches the meninges, forming a tubercle. The tubercle may be dormant for many years. The tubercle then ruptures and releases bacteria into the subarachnoid space causing meningitis. Typically the infection occurs at the base of the brain and causes cranial neuropathies and hydrocephalus from obstruction of cerebrospinal fluid (CSF) flow from fourth ventricle.

Diagnosis can be made with positive PCR test result in the CSF.

Cryptococcosis

Cryptococcus neoformans is a common soil fungus found near roosting sites of birds and pigeons. The clinical picture is very similar to that of TB.

Diagnosis is made with positive CSF latex agglutination test. India ink is not as sensitive.

Progressive multifocal encephalitis

Is caused by JC virus, a human papovavirus.

It causes widespread demyelination in the CNS. Pts present with rapidly progressive dementia followed by focal neurologic signs, including visual changes. Death occurs in less than 6 months. Diagnosis can be made with a positive CSF PCR test result. Treatment is aggressive antiretroviral therapy.

Start empirical treatment for the suspected organism

After the initial CSF profile and head imaging results come back, one should be able to narrow down the diagnosis to one or two organisms. Antibiotics should be started until the definitive test result comes back. Consult an infectious disease specialist.

If pt is HIV positive

Very often in AIDS pts with neurologic symptoms, MRI will show some intracranial abnormalities. The most common causes of intracranial lesions in HIV pt are toxoplasmosis, lymphoma, and PML, in that order.

Toxoplasmosis and lymphoma often have similar MRI findings and it is difficult to distinguish the two clinically.

Standard practice is to treat the pt empirically with anti-toxoplasma meds (sulfadiazine, pyrimethamine, and leucovorin). Repeat MRI 2 to 3 wks after treatment and compare with the first study. If there is a reduction in size/number of lesions, then the diagnosis is toxoplasmosis. If there is no response, then brain biopsy is indicated to diagnose CNS lymphoma.

Do not treat pt with corticosteroids at the same time because it will shrink lymphoma and may confound the diagnosis.

VI
Spinal Cord Disease

Are there any motor or sensory symptoms?

Spinal cord lesion causes loss of motor and/or sensory functions *below the level* of lesion.

Pt may complain of weakness and numbness from waist, chest, or neck down.

Sensory disturbances may involve any modalities including proprioception, for which pt complains of unsteadiness or frequent falls.

Severe back pain points more to epidural abscess or compression fracture.

Pain that radiates to the legs is consistent with caudal equina or conus medullaris syndrome.

Are there any bladder or bowel symptoms?

Urinary incontinence, urgency, retention, and bowel constipation and incontinence support the diagnosis of a spinal cord lesion.

Is sexual dysfunction present?

Ask about loss of libido or erectile dysfunction ranging from impotence to priapism.

Are respiratory symptoms present?

If the lesion involves upper cervical spine (C3, C4, C5), there may be shortness of breath, irregular breathing, and apnea.

Ask about constitutional symptoms

Will help generate a differential diagnosis.

Fever/chill suggests infectious etiology, such as epidural abscess.

Recent evidence of fall or trauma may indicate epidural/subdural hematoma.

Weight loss, night sweats may indicate neoplasm or TB.

Assess vital signs

Irregular breathing and heart rate indicate upper spinal cord involvement.

Assess mental status and cranial nerves

This assessment should be normal. Abnormalities put the lesion above the level of spinal cord.

Document motor exam

If the arms and hands are normal, then the lesion is below T1.

In acute spinal cord injuries, tone and deep tendon reflexes are decreased (spinal shock) and will increase gradually as injuries become chronic.

For caudal equina and conus medullaris, ankle reflex may be absent.

Beevor's sign indicates lesion below T9. Babinski signs are positive.

Perform sensory exam

Check for *sensory level*. The level at which pt begins to feel change in sensation is approximately one to two spinal columns below level of lesion.

Common levels to remember include T10, umbilicus and T4, nipple.

Look for dissociative sensory loss; that is, loss of pain/temperature on one side and loss of proprioception/vibration on the contralateral side. If present, then pt has *Brown-Séquard syndrome*. The lesion is on the side of proprioceptive/vibratory loss.

If pain/temperature is affected but proprioception/vibration is spared, then pt has *anterior cord syndrome*. Conversely, with intact pain/temperature but impaired proprioception/vibration, pt has *posterior cord syndrome*.

If pt has a suspended sensory level (i.e., loss of sensory in arms/upper trunk with normal legs and face), then it is likely *central cord syndrome* in which the lesion is intramedullary (within the spinal cord) at the center expanding outward.

Lower extremity sensory loss in dermatomal distribution is more consistent with caudal equina or conus medullaris syndrome.

Perform rectal exam and check for saddle anesthesia
Saddle anesthesia suggests caudal equina or conus medullaris syndrome.
Rectal tone is decreased in all spinal cord lesions.

Obtain STAT MRI with contrast on the area localized by exam
MRI with contrast is the gold standard. If not available, get CT myelogram.

Acute spinal cord syndromes
The syndromes of spinal cord are classified according to the location and structure involved. They include: complete transection, hemisection, central, anterior, and posterior cord syndromes. Caudal equina and conus medullaris syndromes involve the distal spinal cord and the nerve roots. Mixed findings of upper motor neuron and lower motor neuron lesions are expected.

The most common etiologies are:
- Metastatic carcinoma, with lung, breast, prostate gland, melanoma, and lymphoma most common.
- Spinal cord infarction can be caused by occlusion of anterior spinal artery giving rise to anterior cord syndrome or posterior spinal artery (less common because of two redundant posterior spinal arteries) causing posterior cord syndrome.
- T1 to T4 and L1 level are the vascular watershed area and are susceptible to hypoperfusion injuries. Spinal cord borderzone infarct is most commonly seen in aortic surgery or dissection, when the major radicular artery of Adamkiewicz is compromised.
- Epidural abscess is most often caused by staphylococcus and gram-negative bacilli. Infection can result from hematogenous spread from remote infection or direct extension from psoas abscess, dermal sinus, or decubitus ulcer.
- Transverse myelitis is most often caused by demyelinating disorder such as multiple sclerosis or acute disseminated encephalomyelitis and viral infections such as human T-cell leukemia virus–1, HIV, cytomegalovirus, varicella-zoster virus, and herpes simplex virus.

Admit pt to the hospital
Spinal cord compression is a medical/surgical emergency. If not diagnosed and treated promptly, lifelong paraplegia or quadriplegia will follow.

Start corticosteroids
To decrease inflammation, vasogenic edema, as well as size of any tumor.

Treat the underlying cause
If abscess is found, broad-spectrum antibiotics should be initiated. Consult orthopedic spine or neurosurgery service for drainage.
If infarction, maximize perfusion with adequate blood pressure and volume. If there is evidence of embolization, treat with antiplatelet or anticoagulation therapy.
For transverse myelitis, perform lumbar puncture to establish the cause first and treat with either antivirals or immune modulation therapies.
If there is a tumor, consult neurosurgery and a radiation oncologist.

Initiate physical therapy
After the underlying issue is addressed, initiate physical therapy as soon as possible.

S **Is there a history giving rise to pt's spasticity and muscle spasm?**
Spasticity does not develop acutely. It develops over weeks to months following injury to upper motor neuron pathways. Common causes include:
- Stroke or other brain injury
- Multiple sclerosis
- Cerebral palsy
- Spinal cord injury

O **Perform a general physical exam**
Examine the skin for any breakdown or decubitus ulcer
Palpate bladder for distention as in neurogenic bladder

Perform neurologic exam
Spasticity is best assessed at the elbows, knees, and ankles.
Assess muscle bulk, tone, and strength.
One must differentiate between spasticity and rigidity. They are signs of completely different disease processes. Spasticity results from upper motor neuron (pyramidal tract) lesion such as stroke, whereas rigidity results from extrapyramidal system disease processes such as Parkinson's disease.

The key difference between spasticity and rigidity is that spasticity is *velocity independent* and rigidity is *velocity dependent*. In other words, spasticity may be detected only following the application of fast muscle stretches to the affected limb but is not detected during slow movements. In rigidity, the increased tone is present regardless of how fast you stretch the affected muscle.

Check for clonus and clasp-knife phenomenon
Check Babinski's sign
Check sensory level. Presence of sensory level is pathognomic for spinal cord lesion.

Spasticity and Muscle Spasm
Spasticity has been defined as an increase in muscle tone due to hyperexcitability of the stretch reflex and is characterized by a velocity-dependent increase in tonic stretch reflexes.
It is a common problem affecting over half a million people in the U.S.
The mechanism causing spasticity is very complicated and incompletely understood. Basically, the upper motor system has inhibitory effect on the spinal cord motor neurons. Loss of the inhibitory function results in increased excitation of the neuromuscular system. As the result, the muscles contract excessively and spasticity develops.
Muscle spasms occur when stimulus is applied to the pt below the level of injury. The stimulus can be stretching of muscle, pain, or even light touch. The signal goes to the spinal cord and, without inhibitory input from the upper motor neurons, it triggers the reflex causing the muscle to go into spasm.

Indications for therapy and expectations
Spasticity does not always need to be treated. There are some benefits to spasticity:
- It can serve as a warning mechanism to identify pain or problem in areas where there is no sensation. Many people know when a urinary tract infection is beginning by an increase in muscle spasms.
- Spasticity helps to maintain muscle size and bone strength.
- Spasticity helps to maintain circulation in legs.
- Spasticity can be used to improve certain activities such as transferring from bed to chair or walking with braces.

For these reasons, treatment is usually started only when spasticity interferes with sleep or limits an individual's functional capacity.

Bladder infection and skin breakdown will increase spasms, so treating these conditions will decrease spasms to baseline.

In pt who does not perform regular range of motion exercises, muscles and joints become less flexible and almost any minor stimulation can cause severe spasticity. It is important to get pt involved in long-term physical or occupational therapy.

Consider medications to treat spasticity and spasm

Baclofen and diazepam increase presynaptic (GABAergic) inhibition of Ia afferent fibers, depressing monosynaptic reflex activity. Baclofen also inhibits polysynaptic reflex activity.

Gabapentin also works on GABA receptor and is effective as well.

Tizanidine and clonidine block α2-adrenergic receptors in excitatory interneuronal pathways.

Spasms can also be lessened by inducing weakness of peripheral muscle by dantrolene, which reduces calcium release from sarcoplasmic reticulum.

Consider botulinum toxin injection

Botulinum toxin can also induce weakness of peripheral muscle by creating a presynaptic neuromuscular blockade.

Before giving botulinum toxin, it's important to identify which muscle is involved and to treat. EMG and diagnostic blocks with local anesthetics can help identify which muscles to treat.

Botulinum toxin is effective for approximately 3 months. Pt will need repeated injections at 3-month intervals. Antibodies to botulinum toxin may develop, halting a response.

Consider baclofen pump

Baclofen pump is a device that is implanted subcutaneously in the back. It contains a reservoir of liquid baclofen and delivers a small amount of baclofen directly to the cerebrospinal fluid space.

Because it is delivered directly to the target site, the required dose is extremely small and the therapeutic effect is great. Side effects are very minimal due to small dose.

The baclofen pump is considered the most effective spasticity and spasm treatment by many patients and doctors.

Consider surgical treatment

Rhizotomy is a procedure that involves cutting the posterior roots between the levels of L2 and S2. The posterior roots carry sensory information to the spinal cord. Severing it will abolish the stimulus from entering spinal cord and decreasing spasms.

This procedure has been performed mostly in children with cerebral palsy with severe spasticity of lower extremities. Most pts have good results.

VII

Neuro-Ophthalmology and Otology

S **Ask pt to describe the visual loss**
The first step in evaluating visual disturbance is to determine whether the cause is ophthalmologic or neurologic.
Scotoma (any defect in the visual field) due to macular disease is a "positive" phenomenon. Pt will report seeing a black spot in the visual field or geometric distortion of images.
Scotoma due to neurologic lesion is "negative." Pt will report inability to see. Decreased or change in color perception is common in optic neuritis.
Blurry vision can be reported in both neurologic and ocular diseases.

Did the symptom come and go?
If symptom is transient consider amaurosis fugax, migraine, angle-closure glaucoma, epilepsy, increased intracranial pressure with papilledema, and giant cell arteritis.

Is the symptom unilateral or bilateral?
Causes for monocular visual loss include optic neuritis, anterior ischemic optic neuropathy, central retinal vein/artery occlusion, retinal detachment, vitreous hemorrhage, vasculitis.
For bilateral visual loss causes include optic neuritis (rare), strokes, pituitary apoplexy, optic nerve drusen, toxic, metabolic, and nutritional neuropathies.

Is there any condition that can worsen the symptom?
With optic neuritis, pt may exhibit Uhthoff phenomenon, which is worsening of vision with exertion or following a hot bath.
Visual loss with bright light is seen in retinal disease such as cone dystrophy or vascular disease with poor blood perfusion to the eye.

Is there a history of optic neuritis or other neurologic symptoms?
If there is previous episode of optic neuritis or history of focal weakness and numbness, dizziness, and diplopia, then it is very likely that pt has multiple sclerosis.

Is there pain in the eyes?
Optic neuritis, glaucoma, and pituitary apoplexy are usually associated with eye pain. Vascular causes are not painful. Headache following visual loss is typical for migraine. Headache preceding visual loss is seen in giant cell arteritis.

O **Check and note visual acuity in both eyes**
In optic neuritis, visual acuity is usually severely impaired, > 20/200.

Check color perception
Use color plate to look for dyschromatopsia (↓ color perception) in each eye.

Check visual field
Ask pt to count fingers in all four quadrants with each eye.
If there is visual field defect in both eyes (e.g., homonymous hemianopsia or quadrantanopsia), then the lesion is distal to optic chiasm (optic tract, lateral geniculate body, optic radiation, or occipital lobe).
Compressive lesion at optic chiasm may cause bitemporal hemianopsia or monocular blindness in one eye with partial temporal anopsia in the other eye (von Willebrand knee).

Check for afferent pupillary defect (APD)
The afferent pathway in pupillary response is CN2 and the efferent pathway is CN3. In APD, the affected eye does not constrict to light directly; however, it constricts when the light is shined on the other healthy eye.

Perform funduscopic exam
Papillitis is swelling of the optic disk with blurred and elevated disk margin. Papillitis is difficult to differentiate from papilledema. History will help.

Hemorrhage is seen in anterior ischemic optic neuropathy and central retinal vein and artery occlusion (cherry red spot).

If the lesion is far away from the nerve head (retrobulbar neuritis), the disk may appear normal.

If pt has had previous optic neuritis, the optic disk may appear atrophic and pale.

Perform MRI of brain with and without contrast if lesion is neurologic

Sometimes optic neuritis can be visualized directly on the MRI. Characteristic finding is increased signal on T2-weighted image and enhancement following IV contrast.

MRI evidence of areas of demyelination is diagnostic of multiple sclerosis (MS). Strokes, pituitary apoplexy, and tumors are also diagnosed with MRI.

Perform lumbar puncture in optic neuritis

Cerebrospinal fluid (CSF) should be sent for cell count, glucose, protein, MS panel, Venereal Disease Research Laboratory testing.

Usually CSF will show lymphocyte pleocytosis with elevated protein.

Optic neuritis

More common in young female population (20 to 45 yrs of age, male:female ratio = 1:2)

Optic neuritis is often the first sign of MS, although it can also occur as a stand-alone disease. Other causes of optic neuritis include Lyme disease, syphilis, tuberculosis, viruses such as HIV, hepatitis B virus, cytomegalovirus, herpes simplex virus.

Optic neuritis is *inflammation* of the optic nerve. It should be differentiated from other *optic neuropathies* that may have similar presentation:
- Anterior ischemic optic neuropathy: Due to infarction of optic nerve from posterior ciliary artery occlusion. The vascular lesion can be due to atherosclerosis, diabetes, or vasculitis.
- Compressive optic neuropathy: Masses in or near the orbit (e.g., cavernous sinus, ethmoid, and sphenoid sinus) can compress the nerve and cause infarction. Chronic elevated ICP can also damage the optic nerve as in pseudotumor cerebri.
- Toxic and nutritional optic neuropathy: EtOH, methanol, tobacco, isoniazid, hydroxyquinolines, and vitamin B_{12} deficiency.

Consult ophthalmology immediately if evidence of ocular disease

Glaucoma, retinal vessel occlusion, and hemorrhage need to be dealt with immediately.

Treat optic neuritis with high dose corticosteroid

Start Solumedrol 1 g IV Q 24 hrs for 3 to 5 days.

Do not treat with PO dose because it may increase recurrence of optic neuritis.

Start GI prophylaxis and potassium supplement. Monitor blood glucose.

Inform pt of the prognosis

Pt has an approximate 75% chance of having a complete or near-complete recovery of visual function after few weeks.

If MRI is normal, there is a 20% chance that pt will develop MS within 10 yrs.

If MRI shows one or more demyelinating lesions, the chance of pt developing MS is 56% over the next 10 yrs.

Male gender and absence of eye pain are associated with better prognosis.

S **Does the pt have symptoms of cavernous sinus involvement?**
The classic symptoms of cavernous sinus involvement include:
- Diplopia
- Facial numbness
- Orbital pain or frontal headache

How long have the symptoms been present?
The time course aides in establishing the differential diagnosis
- Sudden onset (seconds to minutes): thrombosis, rupture of aneurysm
- Subacute (hours to days): infection
- Chronic progressive (weeks to months): tumor, aneurysm
- Recurrent: autoimmune, inflammatory

Screen for any constitutional symptoms
Recent dental work followed by fever suggests infection.
Weight loss/night sweats suggest neoplasm.

Perform a general physical exam
Vital signs
Examine the face and look for signs of furuncle, abscess, open wounds.
Check the eye for chemosis, proptosis, and periorbital edema.
Auscultate the forehead and orbits for bruits, which are highly suggestive of internal carotid artery (ICA) fistula.
Check neck for stiffness, and Kernig sign.

Perform a neurologic exam
Carefully compare pupillary size and light reaction on both sides.
Carefully assess extraocular movement.
Check for facial sensation, especially V1 and V2 distribution of trigeminal nerve.

Obtain brain imaging with thin cuts through cavernous sinus
CT is indicated if there is history of trauma. Otherwise, MRI with/without contrast is preferred. They will also show any mass or infection in the paranasal sinuses and orbits.
Order MRA if aneurysm and thrombosis are suspected. It may show decreased or absent flow in the cavernous portion of carotid artery.
Conventional cerebral angiogram is still the gold standard for vascular lesions. Order if MRA is not conclusive.

Anatomy of cavernous sinus
Cavernous sinus is a *venous sinus* space comprised of dural matter.
It receives venous blood from superior and inferior ophthalmic veins and drains via the sphenoparietal sinus, the superior petrosal sinus, the basilar plexus (which drains to the inferior petrosal sinus), and the pterygoid plexus.
The right and left cavernous sinuses are connected by circular sinus. So a disease process can spread from one side to the other and cause bilateral symptoms.

The structures that go through cavernous sinus include:
1. Internal carotid artery
2. CN3
3. CN4
4. CN5 ophthalmic and maxillary divisions (V1 and V2)
5. CN6

Involvement of CN3, CN4, and CN6 causes diplopia.
Involvement of CN5 causes pain and facial numbness.
ICA aneurysm can compress the adjacent cranial nerves. When the aneurysm ruptures, the arterial blood is dumped directly into the venous circulation (i.e., fistula). Proptosis and chemosis develop immediately.
Superior orbital fissure (SOF) *syndrome* is very similar to cavernous sinus thrombosis. Structures that go through SOF include CN3, CN4, CN5 ophthalmic division, CN6, and superior ophthalmic vein. The differential diagnosis is similar with trauma being more common in SOF.

Etiologies of cavernous sinus syndrome
Tumor: meningiomas can arise from the dural tissue. Neurofibromas can arise from the nerve itself. Pituitary adenoma and nasopharyngeal carcinoma can invade the cavernous sinus by local extension. Metastasis from lung and breast is also possible.
Thrombosis
- Often the result of infection in the adjacent paranasal sinuses or orbits. CSF is normal unless the infection spread to the meninges.
- Can also be caused by hypercoagulable state.

Inflammatory diseases
- *Tolosa Hunt syndrome*: idiopathic granulomatous disease of cavernous sinus. Pt presents with painful ophthalmoplegia. Diagnosis is made clinically with elevated ESR and MRI finding of increased signal in cavernous sinus.
- Sarcoidosis

Carotid aneurysm and fistula
Trauma

Treat the underlying cause
In case of tumor, start pt on steroids and obtain neurosurgical consult.
If aneurysm and fistula, the preferred treatment is by interventional radiology to place coils, balloon, or glues to occlude the lumen.
In case of thrombosis, admit pt to the hospital and start heparin. The cause of thrombosis will need to be established. (See chapter on venous thrombosis.)
In case of infection, start pt on appropriate antibiotics. In pts with evidence of furuncle, the most likely organism is *Staphylococcus aureus*. In diabetic or immunocompromised pts, fungi and opportunistic organisms must be ruled out.
In case of inflammatory disease such as Tolosa-Hunt or orbital pseudotumor, treat with prednisone 1 mg/kg/day. The length of therapy varies by pt. If symptoms do not improve after 2 days, a biopsy may be needed to rule out other causes.

S **How do the images of double vision appear?**
Double vision is caused by the misalignment of the two eyes. The pattern of the images is the key to find out which cranial nerve is involved.
On primary gaze, if the double images are
- Diagonal: CN3 palsy
- Vertical: CN4 palsy
- Horizontal: CN6 palsy

Is the double vision persistent with closure of one eye or the other?
If yes, the most likely diagnosis is psychogenic conversion disorder or malingering. It's very rare for ocular or CNS disease to cause monocular diplopia.

What makes the double vision better and what makes it worse?
CN6: better when viewing near objects and worse when viewing far objects.
CN4: better by looking up (chin tuck) and by tilting the head away from the affected eye to compensate for the hypertropia and extorsion.
CN3: worse when looking at near objects and better when looking at distant objects, because convergence and accommodation are impaired.

Is glare in bright light present?
Pupil dilatation (in CN3 palsy) causes glare or discomfort in bright light.

Is there droopy eyelid?
The ptosis is due to weakness of the levator palpebrae muscle, which is innervated by CN3.

Is there pain?
Severe headache and orbital pain may sometimes accompany the CN3 palsy if it is caused by diabetes. Tumors, aneurysm, and central causes do not cause pain.

Is there a history of recent head trauma?
CN4 is the most commonly injured cranial nerve in head trauma, probably due to its long course and thin caliber, making it susceptible to shear injury.

Are there any other focal neurologic symptoms?
The presence of other focal neurologic symptoms (hemi-weakness and sensory loss) is consistent with lesion in the brainstem (i.e., midbrain or pons).

Observe position of eyes on primary gaze
In CN3 palsy the eye will be in a "down and out" position due to actions of intact lateral rectus and superior oblique muscles. Also look for ptosis.
In CN4 palsy, the eyes may look normal or may show hypertropia and extorsion, which may be difficult to appreciate. Pt often has a head tilt away from the side of lesion.
In CN6 palsy, the eyes may appear normal or one eye may deviate laterally.

Check extraocular muscles (EOMs)
Note the percentage of eye movements in all four directions.
If no appreciable EOM defect is noted, ask pt to look and follow your finger, test all directions and at the same time have pt tell you whether diplopia is better or worse:
- In CN6 palsy, diplopia will be worse when looking laterally toward the side of affected eye. The diplopia should resolve when looking away from the side of affected eye.
- In CN4 palsy, diplopia will be worse when looking down and away from the affected side. It will be better or resolve when looking up and toward the side of lesion.
- CN3 palsy is the easiest to tell because of concomitant ptosis. The diplopia is better when looking down and toward the affected side.

Presence of internuclear ophthalmoplegia (INO) suggests lesion in medial longitudinal fasciculus (MLF) and is usually seen with multiple sclerosis or small pontine tumor and infarct.

Horizontal gaze palsy (both eyes unable to move to one side) suggests lesion either in CN6 *nucleus or paramedian pontine reticular formation* (PPRF), which are within brainstem and seen with strokes, tumor, and multiple sclerosis.

Combination of gaze palsy and INO is called $1^{1}/_{2}$ syndrome which is caused by lesion in both MLF and CN6 nucleus.

Check pupil light reaction and accommodation

CN3 has both autonomic and motor function. The parasympathetic fibers are on the outside and oculomotor fibers are inside.

Compression of CN3 will affect the outside first, so pupillary reaction is impaired before ocular paresis and ptosis. The most common causes are posterior communicating artery aneurysm and tumor.

- A "pupil-sparing CN3 palsy" (i.e., ptosis and ocular paresis with intact pupil) indicate lesion limited to the inner portion of the nerve. The most common etiology is microvascular infarct from diabetes.

Presence of afferent pupillary defect (APD) indicates optic nerve dysfunction and is most commonly seen in multiple sclerosis.

Examine the fundi and look for optic nerve papillitis or atrophy, which may be a sign of previous multiple sclerosis attack. Papilledema goes with raised ICP, which may present with CN6 palsy. Look at the retina for signs of diabetes and hypertension.

Complete remainder of neurologic exam

Stupor and coma may be sign of herniation from intracranial pressure.
Look for signs of myasthenia gravis or Guillain-Barré syndrome (GBS), which may present with diplopia/EOM palsy.
Lateralizing finding may indicate stroke in the brainstem.
Neck stiffness may be sign of subarachnoid hemorrhage or meningitis.
Facial pain and numbness may indicate cavernous sinus involvement.

Diplopia

Diplopia can be caused by lesions in the following structures/etiologies listed from most peripheral to central
- Extraocular muscles: orbital fracture with entrapment, thyroid disease, myositis
- Neuromuscular junction: myasthenia gravis, Lambert-Eaton, botulism
- Cranial nerves: CN3, CN4, and CN6 leave the brainstem, enter the subarachnoid space, go through some bony structures into cavernous sinus, and then enter orbits. Any lesion (subarachnoid hemorrhage, meningitis, tumor, aneurysm, trauma, pressure) along the course can cause CN damage. GBS and diabetes damage the myelin/nerve directly.
- Brainstem: Infarct, multiple sclerosis, tumor, and hemorrhage are likely causes. Because brainstem is a packed place, other focal neurologic signs are expected.

Admit pt to hospital

Ocular palsy can be initial sign of serious disease. Interns and junior residents should admit the pt for further observation.

Consider further workup and treatment

Depending on the differential diagnosis, CT, MRI, angiogram, and lumbar puncture may be considered. Treatment will depend on the diagnosis.

S **Does the pt complain of symptoms of Horner syndrome?**
Most cases of Horner syndrome are found incidentally; however, pts may complain of droopy eyelid and dry half of face.

Are there any associated neurologic symptoms?
The following symptoms may help with narrowing the differential diagnosis:
- Headache: migraine or cluster headache
- Facial pain: trigeminal neuralgia
- The 4 Ds—dysarthria, dysphagia, dizziness, diplopia—brainstem lesions
- Neck pain: cervical spine lesion

Are there any systemic or constitutional symptoms?
Fever, cough, weight loss, night sweat may suggest cancer (e.g., Pancoast tumor), TB, sarcoidosis.

Is there any history of trauma to the head or neck?
Any injury, especially to the neck, may cause Horner syndrome.

Ask for any photo identification such as driver's license
Sometimes when the ptosis is subtle, it will be helpful to see an old picture to see whether there is a change from before.

Perform a general physical and neurologic exam
The signs of Horner syndrome are:
- Ptosis
- Miosis
- Anhidrosis

Estimate percentage of lid droop (e.g., 100% would be complete eye closure).
Bring the pt to a dark room. The anisocoria is easier to see in dim conditions.
Record the actual pupil size in millimeter with and without light.
Compare how well the pupils dilate. In Horner syndrome the affected pupil will react and accommodate, but should dilate slower than the normal one because it lacks the pull from dilator muscle.
Pay close attention to extraocular movements. If extraocular muscles are affected, then pt may have ptosis from CN3 palsy, not Horner syndrome.
Feel the facial skin. In warm and humid conditions, anhidrosis sometimes can be seen and felt. However in most cases it is not appreciated on exam.
- Anhidrosis involving entire half face localizes the lesion to the common carotid artery.
- Anhidrosis involving medial forehead and nose localizes the lesion distal to the carotid bifurcation.

Auscultate lung for any areas of decreased breath sound.
Palpate cervical and clavicular lymph nodes.

Horner syndrome

Horner syndrome is not a diagnosis. It is the manifestation of underlying disease processes that interrupt the sympathetic nerve supply to the eye.
The sympathetic innervation to the eye is made up by three neurons:
- First-order neuron: The fibers arise from the posterolateral hypothalamus, descend ipsilaterally through the brainstem and cervical spinal cord and synapse with the second-order neurons at T2 level.
- Second-order neuron: These are the preganglionic sympathetic fibers. They exit the spinal cord, travel in the sympathetic chain to the superior cervical ganglion next to bifurcation of common carotid artery, and synapse with the third-order neurons.
- Third-order neuron: These are the postganglionic sympathetic fibers. They leave the superior cervical ganglion and branch off into fibers supplying the facial sweat glands, pupillary dilator muscle, and Müller muscle (which elevate eyelid).

Etiologies of Horner syndrome depend on which neuron is affected:
- First-order neuron: stroke, syrinx, brain and spinal cord tumors, spinal cord trauma, multiple sclerosis, syphilis
- Second-order neuron: Pancoast tumor, trauma to brachial plexus, dissection or aneurysm of aorta, common carotid, subclavian arteries
- Third-order neuron: internal carotid artery dissection/aneurysm, cluster/migraine headache, herpes zoster, retro-orbital tumor/hematoma, cavernous sinus lesions

Establish that pt has Horner syndrome with 2% cocaine eye solution

Often physical exam finding are subtle and the presence of Horner is dubious. In such cases, give pt 2 drops of 2% cocaine solution to each eye.
Cocaine inhibits the *reuptake* of norepinephrine in the synaptic cleft. The excess norepinephrine will cause the normal pupil to dilate.
The pupil with Horner syndrome has less norepinephrine in the synapse because of decreased release from denervated presynaptic neuron (it doesn't matter whether the lesion is in first-, second-, or third-order neuron). It will not dilate to the same degree as the normal pupil.
Examine the pupil 40 minutes after instillation of the drops. If anisocoria persists, then Horner syndrome is confirmed.

Determine pre- vs. post-ganglionic lesion with 1% hydroxyamphetamine solution

Hydroxyamphetamine causes *release* of norepinephrine from the post-ganglionic third-order neurons into the synapse.
If the lesion is in the third-order neuron, then the damaged neuron won't have enough norepinephrine to be released. The pupil will dilate less than the normal eye.
If the lesion is in the first- or second-order neuron, then the intact third-order neuron will be able to release the ample stored amount of norepinephrine. The pupil will dilate equally or greater than the normal eye.
Be sure to do the hydroxyamphetamine test at least 48 hrs after the cocaine test for an accurate result.

Order the appropriate imaging study and treat the underlying cause

Depending on the localization and differential diagnosis, obtain MRI, CT, angiogram, ultrasound or x-ray on the area of interest.

What does the pt mean by "dizzy"?
Dizziness is a very nonspecific term. Have pt specify what he/she feels exactly.
Dizziness can be divided into the following four categories:
- Vertigo: a sensation of rotation, spinning movement of environment or self. Pt often describes "room spinning."
- Presyncope: a sensation of fainting or passing out.
- Dysequilibrium: a sensation of imbalance while standing or walking with no abnormal sensation in the head.
- Other sensations: floating, giddiness, or other descriptions not covered by the previous categories.

In this chapter, focus will be on vertigo because it is the most common type of dizziness neurologists are asked to evaluate. The most important question to answer: is the vertigo central or peripheral?

What makes the symptom better and what makes it worse?
Peripheral vertigo is often worse with head turning and movement. It is better if pt keeps head still.

Is there nausea and vomiting?
Both central and peripheral vertigo can cause nausea and vomiting. Peripheral vertigo tends to cause more severe nausea and vomiting and pt appears sicker.
If there is no complaint of nausea and vomiting, then pt likely does not have vertigo but some other type of dizziness.

Are there associated neurologic symptoms?
It is rare to have vertigo as the only symptom if pt has a CNS lesion. Ask about visual changes, dysarthria, dysphagia, weakness, and numbness. If pt answers "yes" to any question, then the cause is likely to be central.
Deafness is almost never due to central lesion. If pt has decreased hearing or ear stuffiness, think about Ménière or other inner ear disease.
Ataxia and fall are present in both central and peripheral vertigo. Fall is to the side of lesion.

Carefully perform eye exam
Check extraocular muscles. If abnormal, then pt must have central vertigo.
Observe the nystagmus closely. Nystagmus is defined by the direction of the fast phase.
- In peripheral vertigo:
  - Nystagmus is unidirectional with rotatory component.
  - Direction of nystagmus is away from the affected labyrinth.
  - Nystagmus is more prominent when pt is symptomatic and absent or more subtle when pt does not have vertigo.
  - Nystagmus goes away with visual fixation on an object.
- In central vertigo:
  - Nystagmus is bidirectional with or without rotatory component.
  - Pure vertical nystagmus is consistent with central vertigo.
  - Nystagmus is prominent even when pt doesn't have symptom.
  - Nystagmus is worse with visual fixation.

Examine the ears
Compare hearing on both sides with 256-or 512-Hz tuning fork.
Examine both tympanic membranes.

Complete the neurologic exam to look for evidence of central lesions
Check for focal weakness, sensory deficits, differences in tones and reflexes, Babinski signs.
Finger-nose and gait ataxia are seen in both central and peripheral vertigo.

Perform Dix-Hallpike maneuver
Quickly move the pt from sitting to supine position with head dropped 30° below end of the table and rotate the head 40° to one side. Ask pt about dizziness and observe for nystagmus for approximately 30 seconds. Repeat the test with head rotated to the other direction. If during the maneuver pt's vertigo and nystagmus are reproduced, then the test result is positive.
A positive Hallpike test establishes the diagnosis of benign paroxysmal positional vertigo (BPPV).

Consider electronystagmogram
Usually not necessary if examiner is experienced in evaluating nystagmus. It records the patterns of nystagmus with gazes, Hallpike, and caloric testing.

Consider brain MRI
Only if central cause of vertigo is suspected.

Vertigo
Vertigo can be caused by lesion/disorder anywhere in the vestibular pathway from most peripheral to central
- Vestibular end organs (cochlear, semicircular canal, labyrinth): BPPV, trauma, Ménière, aminoglycoside toxicity.
- Vestibular division of CN8: vestibular neuronitis, herpes zoster, cerebellopontine angle tumors such as acoustic neuroma.
- Vestibular nuclei in the brainstem and connections to the cerebellum: stroke, tumors, infection, multiple sclerosis, basilar migraine.
- Connections from cerebellum to lateral thalamus to medial temporal lobe: seizures, tumor, trauma, episodic ataxia (a hereditary potassium channelopathy).

If central vertigo, establish the cause and treat the underlying lesion.
For peripheral vertigo, treat symptomatically
Start with meclizine 25 mg PO Q 8 hrs PRN or diazepam 5 mg PO Q 4 hrs PRN. Both treat vertigo effectively. Diazepam has more side effects (such as sedation), so start with meclizine first.
Acetazolamide is effective for treating familial episodic ataxia and Ménière disease by reducing endolymph production. Pt should also reduce salt intake.
Prescribe anti-emetics if severe nausea and vomiting.

For BPPV, perform Epley maneuver
Begin with Hallpike maneuver to the side that reproduces vertigo. After 20 seconds, turn the head 90° to the other side. After 20 seconds, turn the pt's body to the side while rotating the head so it is parallel to the ground. After 20 seconds, turn head to face ground. After 20 seconds, return pt to sitting position while maintaining the same head position. The pt is to remain at least 45° upright for the next 48 hrs. The maneuver can be repeated in 1 to 2 weeks if vertigo does not resolve.
It has > 90% success rate for treating BPPV. It works by repositioning the blocked canalith.

# VIII
Neuromuscular Disease

S

What symptoms does the pt complain of?
Symptoms can be nonspecific, such as generalized fatigue and exercise intolerance.
Pt may have focal weakness, complaining of weakness in one arm or leg.
In approximately half of pts, the initial complaint is double vision and drooping eyelids from weakness of extraocular muscles and levator palpebrae.
Approximately 10% present initially with facial weakness, difficulty chewing, swallowing, and speaking.

Are there respiratory symptoms, such as shortness of breath?
If yes, pt will need to be monitored closely because diaphragm weakness and respiratory failure can develop rapidly (within hours).

Does anything improve the symptoms?
Hallmark of myasthenia gravis (MG) is that the weakness improves with rest. Usually pt starts out the day feeling normal and as the day wears on, the weakness increases. Weakness is also increased with repetitive use of the affected muscle group.

Are there any symptoms of thyroid dysfunction?
Hyperthyroidism and hypothyroidism are seen in approximately 5% of MG pts. Symptoms include weight loss/gain, diarrhea/constipation, and heat/cold intolerance.

For pts with existing diagnosis and treatment of MG, ask about cholinergic symptoms

Pts with a history of MG may present with either MG exacerbation or cholinergic crisis from too much cholinesterase inhibitor. The two conditions have the same presentation and are difficult to distinguish. Clues that suggest cholinergic crisis include presence of salivation, lacrimation, urinary incontinence, diarrhea, GI upset/hypermotility, and emesis (SLUDGE).

O

Assess vital signs and check forced vital capacity
Pay particular attention to respiration. Is the breathing labored? Is the pt using accessory muscles?
Vital capacity should be checked on all pts suspected or diagnosed with MG.
Alternatively, one can have pt count after taking single deep breath. Ability to reach 20 usually correlates with vital capacity of > 1.5 L.

Assess extraocular muscles (EOMs) and strengths of eye opening and closure
Any EOMs can be affected. Both levator palpebrae (opens eyelids) and orbicularis oculi (closes eyelids) can be affected at the same time.
The presence of normal pupillary response in the face of weakness of EOMs, levator, and orbicularis oculi, is virtually diagnostic of MG.
Check for fatigability of the EOMs and levator by having pt look upward for 60 seconds.

Perform motor exam
Note the degree and pattern on weakness.
Muscle tone is normal to low.
Muscle bulk should be normal unless in chronic MG. There should not be pain on palpation of muscles. If present, consider diagnosis of myositis.
Reflexes are usually preserved. If they are absent then consider diagnosis of peripheral neuropathy such as Guillain-Barré syndrome (GBS).
Check for fatigability by exercising pt (e.g., squats, stair climbing).

Perform edrophonium (Tensilon) test
Mix 10 mg of edrophonium in 10 cc of normal saline in a syringe. Have 1 vial of atropine available at bedside. Connect pt to a cardiac monitor. Place peripheral IV access.

Choose a muscle affected and note baseline degree of weakness with maximum effort.
Inject a test dose of 1 mg edrophonium through IV. If the dose is tolerated then push the rest over 1 minute.
Re-examine that particular muscle. Presence of *marked* improvement is diagnostic of MG. A subjective or marginal improvement is inconclusive. A negative test result does not necessarily rule out MG.
Risks of the test include cardiac bradycardia, arrhythmia, and hypotension due to excess acetylcholine (ACh).

Obtain nerve conduction study with repetitive stimulation
The amplitude of compound muscle action potential (CMAP) will rapidly decrease after exercise if pt has MG. This is diagnostic of MG.

Send serum anti-ACh receptor antibody
This test has good sensitivity and very high specificity. It is found in 90% of patients with generalized MG and 60% of pts with ocular MG.

Myasthenia Gravis
Autoimmune disorder with autoantibodies directed toward the postsynaptic acetylcholine receptor at neuromuscular junctions in skeletal muscles.
Prevalence is approximately 14 per 100,000. It affects pts of both genders and all age groups. Mean age of onset is 28 for female and 42 for male.
The differential diagnosis includes botulism, Lambert-Eaton syndrome (LES), GBS, organophosphate poisoning, myositis, progressive external ophthalmoplegia (PEO), thyrotoxicosis with myopathy.
LES is very similar to MG. In LES, the autoantibody is directed toward calcium channels on presynaptic motor nerve, causing decreased release of ACh. Unlike MG, LES pts improve with exercise as more ACh accumulates in the cleft and Ca^{2+} accumulates in the nerves.

If pt is in MG crisis, admit to ICU and start immune modulation therapy
Rule out cholinergic crisis first. Perform edrophonium test if unclear.
With vital capacity < 15 mL/kg, pt should be intubated.
Either intravenous immunoglobulin or plasmapheresis can be used (see GBS, p. 84).

Start anticholinesterase drug
Start pyridostigmine 60 mg PO TID. Titrate up slowly to control symptoms.

Obtain CT scan of the chest and consider thymectomy
Thymoma occurs in 15% of pts with MG and lymphofollicular hyperplasia of the thymic medulla in 65%.
Thymectomy should be done in pts found to have thymoma.
Thymectomy is also recommended for pts younger than 55 yrs of age who do not respond well or require higher dose of medication.
Remission rate after thymectomy is 35% in non-tumor pts. Another 50% will have significant improvement. The response to thymectomy is observed after approximately 3 yrs.

Consider immunosuppressant medications
For pts who do not respond well to pyridostigmine or thymectomy.
Common agents used are corticosteroids, azathioprine, and cyclosporine.

S — Was there preceding flu-like illness or diarrhea?
Approximately 60% of pts with Guillain-Barré syndrome (GBS) have an antecedent respiratory or gastrointestinal infection 1 to 3 weeks before the onset of symptoms. Less commonly, GBS can follow an immunization or surgical procedure.

Does the pt have any weakness or numbness?
Nonspecific paresthesias and numbness in the hands and toes appear first.
An *ascending weakness* then occurs, starting from the legs and moving to the arms over the course of several days to a week or two.

Does the pt have double vision, difficulty swallowing or speaking?
Cranial nerves are involved frequently, causing diplopia, dysphagia, and dysarthria. When pt has cranial nerve symptoms, it is important to take precautions to prevent aspiration pneumonia (e.g., keep head of bed elevated 45 degrees, NPO, or dysphagia diet).

Does the pt have respiratory symptoms?
GBS often affects the phrenic nerves supplying the diaphragms, causing shortness of breath and CO_2 retention. Those pts need to be monitored closely.

Does the pt have any symptoms of autonomic dysfunction?
Urinary retention or incontinence, loss of sweating or profuse diaphoresis, and facial flushing are common in GBS.

O — Assess the vital signs
Look for bradycardia or tachycardia and fluctuating hypertension and hypotension. These are due to autonomic dysfunction.
Observe respiration. Look for labored breathing and use of accessory respiratory muscles (parasternal, scalene, sternocleidomastoid, trapezius, and pectoralis).

Assess cranial nerve functions
Extraocular muscles, facial muscle strength, and presence of gag reflex.

Perform motor testing
Document strength of each major muscle group. Weakness is usually symmetric. Tone is decreased. Reflex is diminished to absent. Babinski is absent. Gait is impaired.

Check forced vital capacity
Vital capacity is the best object bedside test to monitor pt's respiratory status. Alternatively, ask pt to take deep breath and count quickly. The ability to reach 20 in one breath corresponds to a vital capacity > 1.5 L.

Perform lumbar puncture
Opening pressure should be normally < 20 mm Hg.
Cell count is usually < $10/mm^3$, but can be more, with predominantly lymphocytes. The cell count should return to normal after 2 to 3 days.

Glucose is normal. Protein may be normal the first 3 days but should be elevated afterward for 4 to 6 wks (*albumino-cytologic dissociation*).

Order EMG and nerve conduction study (NCS)
EMG/NCS are diagnostic of GBS. Results may be normal the first few days but afterward will show prolonged F response, distal latency, conduction block, reduced conduction velocity, and reduced compound muscle action potential.
It also has prognostic value. If axonal damage is seen (rather than demyelinating), it portends a poor prognosis for complete recovery.

Guillain-Barré syndrome

It affects children and adults of all ages and both genders. Incidence is estimated at two cases per 100,000 persons per year.

It is caused by autoantibodies attacking the myelin of peripheral nerves, resulting in inflammation and demyelination. The generation of the auto-antibodies is triggered by exposure to certain viral and bacterial antigens.

Campylobacter jejuni, HIV, cytomegalovirus, Epstein-Barr virus, *Mycoplasma pneumoniae*, Lyme disease, and certain vaccines are all associated with GBS.

Miller-Fisher syndrome is a variant of GBS. Pt has ophthalmoplegia, areflexia, and ataxia. Serum antineural antibody, anti-GQ1B, is diagnostic.

The differential diagnosis of GBS includes acute spinal cord disease, myasthenia gravis, tick paralysis, diphtheria, poliomyelitis, porphyria, toxins (botulism, saxitoxin, ciguatoxin, and tetrodotoxin), organophosphate poisoning, and other peripheral neuropathies.

Admit pt to the hospital

GBS is rapidly fatal without intervention if respiratory function is involved.

Vital capacity should be checked Q 4 to 6 hrs in acute illness.

Baseline ABG should be obtained.

Pt with vital capacity < 20 mL/kg should be admitted to ICU.

A vital capacity < 15 mL/kg is an indication for intubation.

Pt with dysphagia or cranial nerve signs should be NPO. Order speech/swallow evaluation before starting PO.

Blood pressure may be labile due to autonomic dysfunction. Treat with IV antihypertensives and pressors if BP is way out of range.

GI ileus sometimes is a problem. Use pro-motility agent and stool softener. Monitor amount of tube feeding.

Start immune modulation therapy

Because the disease is caused by autoantibodies attacking peripheral nerves, the rationale is to remove those antibodies.

Either intravenous immune globulin (IVIG) or plasmapheresis can be used.

IVIG (total 2 g/kg IV divided over 5 days) works slower but is easier and safer to administer.

Plasmapheresis has a quicker response but requires large central line (such as Vas-Cath) and has more serious side effects because large volume of plasma is being exchanged.

Assure and inform pt and pt's family regarding prognosis

GBS has mortality of approximately 3% to 5% even with best treatment. Death is usually due to cardiac arrest and respiratory failure.

Vast majority of pts recover completely. Approximately 10% will have pronounced residual disability.

Recovery usually takes days to weeks. If axonal damage was present, recovery may take months to years.

GBS is monophasic. However, about 5% to 10% will have recurrent or progressive illness. If that is the case, the diagnosis becomes chronic inflammatory demyelinating polyneuropathy.

S **Does the pt complain of weakness?**
Botulism affects both smooth and skeletal muscles. Weakness involves both cranial and peripheral muscles. The weakness progresses from top to bottom and from proximal to distal.
Diplopia and blurred vision occurs first, followed by dysarthria, dysphagia, and dysphonia. Neck, arms, respiratory, lower extremities weakness then occurs in that order.
For infants, symptoms may be poor feeding, lethargy, weak cry, decreased sucking, floppy head, and decreased movements.

Does the pt have any GI symptoms?
For infants, constipation is the most common. Botulism should be first on the differential diagnosis with presentation of a floppy baby with constipation.
For older children and adults, botulism can develop after ingestion of tainted food. Anorexia, nausea, vomiting, diarrhea, and constipation occur within 12 to 36 hrs.

Does the pt have a history of IV drug use?
Clostridium botulinum spore can germinate under anaerobic environment. IV drug users often have abscesses that allow the spores to germinate.

Did the pt eat any home-canned food?
Salsa, baked potato in sealed aluminum foil, cheese sauce, honey, fermented fish, and jalapeno pepper are the most common contaminated sources.

Is there any risk for terrorist threat?
Botulinum toxin is the most potent toxin known and has been used in biologic warfare. It is 100,000 times more toxic than sarin, the organophosphate nerve agent used in the 1995 Tokyo subway terrorist attack that killed 11 and injured more than 5500 people.

O **Assess vital signs**
Especially respiratory rate. Look for signs of accessory muscle use.
Check vital capacity, if less than 20 mL/kg consider intubation.

Check pupillary reaction
Botulism is very difficult to distinguish from myasthenia gravis; however, a careful pupillary exam can establish the diagnosis. In botulism, pupillary light response is absent or diminished. It may still react but is *fatigable*, meaning that the response diminishes with each succeeding light exposure. In MG, pupils are not affected.

Complete remainder of neurologic exam
Ocular exam will show ophthalmoplegia or selective CN3, CN4, CN6 palsies.
Bi-facial palsy with nasal voice is common.
Note the pattern of weakness. Weakness should be symmetric. Proximal muscles are usually more affected more than distal ones.
Deep tendon reflexes should be present but could be absent in severe cases. Muscle tone is decreased. Babinski is negative.
Sensory should be intact. If abnormal consider Guillain-Barré syndrome.

Look for signs of autonomic dysfunction
Orthostatic hypotension, ↓ bowel sounds, bladder distension, dry mouth.

Send off laboratory studies
Send standard labs, chemistry, CBC, urinalysis, ABG tox screen, and CXR
Send a sample of serum, stool, and wound exudate (if present) to the state public health laboratory or Centers for Disease Control (CDC) for bioassay test. (A small sample is injected into mice, if the mice develops botulism then the diagnosis is confirmed. Specific botulinum toxin can be identified through combinations of anti-toxin injections.)

Send stool culture. If *C. botulinum* grows it is also confirmatory of botulism.

Consider nerve conduction study (NCS)
NCS can confirm the diagnosis. Findings include ↓ amplitude of muscle potential and ↑ amplitude with rapid repetitive nerve stimulation.

Botulism
Botulism is rare but important to recognize because early intervention may be life-saving. There are approximately 100 to 200 cases annually in the U.S. Western states (CA, WA, CO, NM, OR) account for more than half of all outbreaks.

Botulism is caused by the exotoxin produced by the gram-positive, anaerobic, spore-forming bacterium *C. botulinum*.

The toxin gets absorbed and enters bloodstream. The toxin then binds irreversibly to the presynaptic nerve terminal of the peripheral nervous system, gets internalized, and cleaves the neuroexocytosis apparatus that releases acetylcholine. The end result is absence of acetylcholine in the nerve terminal causing muscle paralysis and autonomic dysfunction.

There are four ways botulism can occur.
- Foodborne botulism: caused by ingestion of preformed toxin in food
- Wound botulism: Spores in the air reach the wound and germinate under anaerobic condition. The bacteria multiply and produce toxins that are released into bloodstream. GI symptoms are usually absent.
- Infant botulism: Spores enter the gut and germinate under anaerobic conditions. Because the normal flora is absent or under development, *C. botulinum* is allowed to colonize and produce toxins that are absorbed through the gut.
- Adult infectious botulism: Same mechanism as infant botulism. It is rare and usually seen in pts with GI abnormalities such as GI surgery, or long-term antibiotic treatment, which disrupts the normal flora.

Admit pt to ICU for supportive care
Mechanical ventilation for pts with respiratory failure.
Gastric lavage to remove contaminated food.
Cathartic and enema are useful to remove unabsorbed toxins in GI tract. Avoid Mg citrate because Mg can enhance the action of botulinum toxin.

Administer botulinum immunoglobulin
The antitoxin can be obtained from CDC or state public health. It will neutralize circulating toxin and should be given ASAP. The toxin is hand-couriered immediately but may take many hours to get to the pt, depending on the location. Call CDC as soon as clinical diagnosis is made. Do not wait for laboratory results to come back.

If antitoxin is administered, mortality is 10% compared to 46% without treatment.
If antitoxin is administered within 24 hrs, median hospital stay is 10 days compared to 41 days if administered after 24 hrs.

S **What are the common symptoms of peripheral neuropathy?**
Sensory complaints are the most common.
- Pain: burning, lancinating, aching, dysesthesia (uncomfortable paraesthesia), and allodynia (pain with innocuous stimuli such as wearing socks).
- Numbness or reduced sensation.
- Hyperesthesia (increased sensation).
- Loss of proprioceptive sensation resulting in ataxia and frequent falls.

Motor symptoms include weakness, muscle wasting, and cramps.

Obtain detailed medical history and social history
Peripheral neuropathy is usually a manifestation of underlying illness such as diabetes, renal failure, polyarteritis nodosa, systemic lupus erythematosus, Churg-Strauss, hepatitis, HIV, and hypothyroidism.
Alcoholism is the second most common cause of peripheral neuropathy in developed countries (diabetes is the most common).
Vitamin B_{12} deficiency from strict vegetarian diet is another cause of neuropathy.

Is there travel history? Is the pt originally from foreign country?
Worldwide, leprosy is the most common cause of peripheral neuropathy and is caused by *Mycobacterium leprae* endemic in Asia, Africa, and S. America.

Review medication
Isoniazid (due to vitamin B_6 deficiency), vincristine, hydralazine, disulfiram, cisplatin, metronidazole are common drugs that cause neuropathy.

Is there family history of neuropathy or weakness?
Peripheral neuropathy sometimes is hereditary such as Charcot-Marie-Tooth.

Perform general physical exam
Look for signs of systemic illness such as lymphadenopathy, hepatosplenomegaly, anemia, skin lesions, clubbing, Mees' lines (growth arrest bands in nail bed in arsenic poisoning).
Look for signs of long-standing neuropathy with pes cavus, kyphoscoliosis, loss of hair in affected area, ulceration, and Charcot joint.

Perform motor exam
Including the cranial muscles. Note degree and pattern of weakness (symmetric or asymmetric, distal or proximal, and confined to a particular nerve, plexus or root level). Tone is decreased. Deep tendon reflexes are reduced or absent. Toes must be down-going.

Perform detailed sensory exam
Test all sensory modalities: light touch, pinprick, temperature, vibration, and proprioception. Note pattern of sensory loss (symmetric or asymmetric, distal or proximal, and confined to a particular nerve, plexus, or root level).
In patients with loss of proprioception, with eyes closed there may be Romberg sign and finger pseudoathetosis (athetoid movement of fingers as if playing piano).

Order EMG/nerve conduction studies
Confirm the presence of neuropathy.
Distinguish what type of fiber is involved (sensory, motor, or both).
Provide pathophysiology (axonal loss vs. demyelinating).
Provide pattern of involvement (symmetric vs. asymmetric, multifocal).

Consider lab studies
Subsequent lab studies should be tailored to the most likely diagnosis. For most pts, routine labs that should be checked include: fasting glucose, BUN, creatinine, HgbA1c, CBC, liver function tests, urinalysis, vitamin B_{12} level, and thyroid-stimulating hormone.

If indicated, check ESR, anti-nuclear antibodies, cryoglobulin, perform serum and urine protein electrophoresis, check heavy metal and homocystine, anti-gliadin antibody, immunofixation, GM_1 antibody.

Consider lumbar puncture
If polyradiculopathy is suspected, lumbar puncture should be done and sent for glucose, protein, cell count, cytology (lymphoma), Lyme, and cytomegalovirus polymerase chain reaction.
Albuminocytologic dissociation (elevated protein in face of normal cell count) is present in inflammatory neuropathy (Guillain-Barré syndrome [GBS], chronic inflammatory demyelinating polyradioneuropathy [CIDP]).

Consider nerve biopsy
If vasculitis, leprosy, amyloidosis, leukodystrophies, and sarcoidosis are suspected.

Peripheral neuropathy
The peripheral nervous system includes the cranial nerves (except CN2), spinal nerve roots, ganglions, peripheral nerves, and autonomic system.
There are two types of axons: large fiber axons include motor axons and sensory axons that carry vibration and proprioception. Small fiber axons include autonomic axons and sensory axons that carry light touch, pain, and temperature. Neuropathy is often classified as large fiber vs. small fiber.
Neuropathies can be caused by damages at these three levels:
- Axons (axonopathy): With focal injury such as trauma, the axon degenerates distal to the site of injury (Wallerian degeneration). With toxic/metabolic injury, the most distal portions of the axons degenerate first in "dying-back" process. This is because of the fact that axonal transport of nutrients is *length-dependent* (so feet are usually affected first).
- Nerve cell body at motor neuron or dorsal root ganglia (neuronopathy): Because the injury is at the cell body, recovery is often incomplete.
- Myelin (myelinopathy): Damage is usually by inflammation. Because the axon is relatively spared, recovery is usually good. Hereditary abnormalities of myelin can occur and run a slow progressive course.

The most common presentation of peripheral neuropathy is *distal symmetric sensorimotor polyneuropathy* and the differential diagnosis (DDx) includes:
- Diabetes, hypothyroidism, EtOH, vitamin B_{12} deficiency, critical care neuropathy, amyloidosis, HIV, organophosphate/heavy metal poisoning, and drugs such as chemotherapies, colchicines, isoniazid, metronidazole, vitamin B_6, dapsone, phenytoin, lithium, chloroquine, ethambutol, amitriptyline, amiodarone, HAART, gold

For *proximal symmetric motor polyneuropathy*, the DDx includes:
- GBS, CIDP, diabetes mellitus, porphyria, multiple myeloma, macroglobulinemia, monoclonal gammopathy, heavy metal poisoning, diphtheria, Lyme, HIV, chemotherapy

For asymmetric (focal or multifocal) neuropathies, the DDx includes:
- Entrapment (focal compression, myxedema, rheumatoid arthritis, acromegaly, amyloidosis), trauma, vasculitis (systemic lupus erythematosus, polyarteritis nodosa, Sjögren's), diabetes, lead poisoning, leprosy, sarcoidosis, hereditary (Charcot-Marie-Tooth disease, pressure palsies)

In approximately 25% of cases, the etiology for peripheral neuropathy cannot be found.

Identify the cause and treat underlying illness and the symptoms
See other chapters on the treatment of specific peripheral neuropathies.

Does the pt have symptoms of chronic inflammatory demyelinating polyradiculoneuropathy (CIDP)?
Subtle sensory disturbances such as tingling and numbness in the hands and feet may be the initial complaint.
Muscle weakness, *particularly proximal*, may occur. Pt may complain of fatigue, exercise intolerance, difficulty climbing stairs, getting out of chair, and reaching overhead objects.
Distal muscle weakness may manifest as difficulty opening cans and jars, dropping things, easy hand fatigue with writing and typing.
Autonomic nervous system may be affected too. Pt complains of dizziness on standing, palpitation, bladder and bowel retention or incontinence.

Does the pt have any risk factors for developing CIDP?
CIDP often is idiopathic but may be associated with the following illnesses:
- Chronic infections such as HIV, hepatitis B virus, hepatitis C virus.
- Hematologic cancers: such as Hodgkin lymphoma, monoclonal gammopathies (particularly IgM), Waldenstrom macroglobulinemia, myeloma, POEMS syndrome.
- Multiple sclerosis.
- Autoimmune disorders such as systemic lupus erythematosus.
- Inflammatory bowel disease such as Crohn's disease.
- Diabetes mellitus, CIDP may overlap with diabetic peripheral neuropathy.
- Pregnancy, especially during third trimester and in the postpartum period.

Does the pt have history of Guillain-Barré syndrome (GBS)?
CIDP may be considered the chronic form of GBS. If patient has GBS with new or worsening weakness, the diagnosis is likely CIDP.

What is the time course of the symptoms?
By definition CIDP is a chronic disease. It begins insidiously and evolves slowly, either in progressive or stepwise fashion, over months to years. If the symptom evolves over days to weeks, consider GBS as the diagnosis. If the symptom is acute, consider mononeuritis multiplex.

Perform general physical
Pay attention to signs of associated conditions previously mentioned.
Look for cachexia, lymphadenopathy, skin rashes, and hepatosplenomegaly.

Perform motor exam
Bifacial weakness if cranial nerve is involved.
Strength is decreased symmetrically with proximal ≥ distal involvement.
Tone is decreased. Reflexes are diminished, especially at the ankles.
Atrophy and fasciculation may be seen.
Observe gait.

Perform sensory exam
Proprioception and vibration are affected more because its fibers are large and heavily myelinated. Romberg sign will be positive.
Pain and temperature are affected to a lesser degree.
Note the pattern of sensory involvement. Stocking-glove distribution is common.

Send labs
Chemistry panel, CBC, ESR cryoglobulin, anti-nuclear antibodies, serum protein electrophoresis, urine protein electrophoresis, HIV, and vitamin B_{12}.

Perform lumbar puncture

As in GBS, cerebrospinal fluid usually shows cytoalbumin dissociation with elevated protein and normal cells.

Protein is usually between 75 and 200 mg/dL. Occasionally it can reach > 1000 mg/dL and is usually associated with pseudotumor cerebri picture.

Cell count is usually normal but in 10% of cases it may be elevated with predominately lymphocytes.

Order EMG/nerve conduction studies (NCS)

EMG/NCS is the most importance tests in diagnosing neuropathies. NCS shows typical demyelinating pattern with prolonged distal latencies, multifocal conduction block, temporal dispersion of compound muscle action potential, and absent/prolonged F wave latencies.

As the disease progresses without treatment, axonal damage can be detected.

Chronic Inflammatory Demyelinating Polyradiculoneuropathy

The exact incidence of CIDP is unknown but is probably underdiagnosed because most primary care physicians are not familiar with the disease.

Affects all age groups and males slightly more than females.

There are segmental demyelination of peripheral nerves caused by immunologic antibody-mediated reaction along with interstitial and perivascular infiltration of the endoneurium with inflammatory T cells and macrophages.

Differential diagnosis includes GBS, multifocal motor neuropathy, diabetic neuropathy, nutritional neuropathy, toxic neuropathy, metabolic neuropathy, vasculitis neuropathy.

Initiate intravenous immunoglobulin (IVIG)

Infuse total 2 g/kg divided over 4 to 5 days.

Most pts benefit from IVIG and report improvement in strength.

The treatment may need to be repeated in progressive cases or when pt has relapse.

Consider plasmapheresis

Plasmapheresis works by removing auto-antibodies from the body.

The clinical response is seen quicker but lasts shorter as well.

Consider corticosteroids

Unlike GBS, CIDP responds to corticosteroids. Start with 80 to 60 mg/day and gradually taper down to a lowest effective dose.

Consider other immunosuppressants

Azathioprine and/or cyclophosphamide may be added to corticosteroid if response is not optimal.

Initiate physical and occupational therapy

Physical and occupational therapy help with maintaining muscle strength and prevent muscle wasting.

Prognosis

Overall prognosis is good with approximately 80% of pts improving with treatment.

Pts with relapsing disease course do better than those with progressive disease course.

Pt may require treatment for many years. The disease may run its course without requiring additional treatment. It may also progress to severe disability.

S **Ask about the weakness**
Determine the age of onset and the progression. What kind of tasks does the pt have difficulty with? What are the provoking or relieving factors? What is the temporal course, constant or episodic?

Obtain detailed family history
Many muscle diseases are hereditary. If the family history is positive and pt is young, consider muscular dystrophies or congenital myopathies.

O **Perform general physical exam**
Observe for any skin rash, especially heliotrope rash on the nose, cheek, forehead, fingernail, and extensor surfaces of elbows, knuckles, and knees.
Look for signs of metabolic disorders, malignancy, infections, and malnutrition.

Perform neurologic exam
The goal of the neurologic exam is to determine where the weakness stems from—muscle, neuromuscular junction, peripheral nerve, spinal cord, or brain.
Spinal and brain (CNS) causes of weakness can be ruled out with normal muscle strength, normal or decreased reflex, normal tone, and nonfocal involvement (i.e., not hemi- or para-paretic).
Peripheral neuropathy is ruled out with a normal sensory, reflex, and tone.
Neuromuscular junction (NMJ) disease can be ruled out by absence of fatigability.
Characteristics of muscle disease include: weakness, atrophy, normal to low reflex, proximal/distal gradient, and possibly symmetry and tenderness.

Obtain laboratory studies
Chem 12, CBC, creatine kinase (CK), aldolase, erythrocyte sedimentation rate, rheumatoid factor, anti-nuclear antibodies, anti-Jo1, urine myoglobinuria.
Obtain ECG because in dermatomyositis (DM) and polymyositis (PM) there is involvement of myocardium as well.
Eosinophilia on CBC may be clue to parasitic myositis.

Order EMG/nerve conduction studies (NCS) and consider muscle biopsy
To confirm the presence of myopathy and to rule out psychogenic, neuropathic, or NMJ diseases. It also determines the best site for muscle biopsy.
Muscle biopsy will be required if diagnosis remains unclear after EMG/NCS.

A **Myopathies and myositis**
They all have the same manifestation—weakness. The important things to keep in mind when generating differential diagnosis are (1) age, (2) clinical course, (3) family history. Below are the common myopathies and myositis.

Dermatomyositis
A relatively common disease affecting all age groups, females > males.
Cause is unknown but probably involves autoimmune process. There is high association with Sjögren's, systemic lupus erythematosus, CREST, and rheumatoid arthritis.
Characterized by acute to subacute progressive and painless weakness of the proximal muscles, especially the hips, thighs and shoulders.
Heliotrope rash involves many body parts, especially extensor surfaces.

Polymyositis
Same as DM except it affects mainly adults and lacks the skin feature.

Inclusion body myositis (IBM)
Affects pts in middle or late adult life with males affected more than females.
Unlike DM and PM, IBM affects distal muscles first. Flexor pollicis longus (distal thumb flexion) involvement is common. It is progressive, painless, and can be asymmetric.

CK is normal or only slightly elevated. Definitive diagnosis requires muscle biopsy, which shows characteristic inclusion bodies.
No effective treatment exists. Disease is progressive and prognosis is poor.

Infectious polymyositis
Parasite: trichinosis, toxoplasmosis, cysticercosis, echinococcosis, trypanosomiasis.
Viral agents include HIV, human T-cell leukemia virus–1, and Coxsackie virus.

Drug-induced myopathies
AZT, EtOH, statins, fibrates

Congenital myopathies
Central core disease: present as floppy infants at birth. Weakness is nonprogressive.
  Type 1 muscle fibers have central pallor consisted of myofibrillar disarray and absence of mitochondria. Defect is in ryanodine receptor gene (involved in calcium channel function).
Nemaline myopathy: present as floppy infant at birth. Weakness is nonprogressive.
  Type 1 muscle fibers consist of multiple dense "threads." Defect is in tropomyosin gene.
Centronuclear myopathy: onset 5 to 30 years of age. X-linked with defect in myotubularin gene. Pt has oculofacial and distal muscle weakness.

Metabolic myopathies
Glycogen storage: acid maltase deficiency, McArdle, Pompe's, Forbes-Cori
Hyperthyroidism and hypothyroidism, corticosteroid myopathy, critical care myopathy, Addison's disease, hyperaldosteronism, hypoparathyroidism, vitamin D deficiency

Periodic paralysis
A group of hereditary disorders caused by ion channel diseases (channelopathies) that manifest as episodic muscle weakness precipitated by strenuous exercise or rich carbohydrate meal. It affects children and young adults.
Hypokalemic periodic paralysis is the most common and caused by defect in Ca^{2+} channel. Many other Ca^{2+}, Na^+, and Cl^- channelopathies also exist.
Diagnosis of hypokalemic periodic paralysis is made by detecting low potassium level during attack. In normal state, attacks can be induced by glucose challenge.
Treatment is daily administration of 5–10 g of KCl.

P **For dermatomyositis and polymyositis, start corticosteroid**
For acute/severe cases, start methylprednisolone 1 g IV QD for 3 days followed by maintenance prednisone. For less severe cases start prednisone 1 mg/kg.
After pt shows response (improvement in strength and decrease in serum CK), the steroid can be tapered to approximately 5–20 mg QD or QOD.
Pt will need to be maintained on steroid for months to 1 to 2 years.
Consider azathioprine, methotrexate, and intravenous immunoglobulin if no response to steroid.
Overall prognosis is good. Pts usually respond well to therapy.

Screen for cancer if dermatomyositis or polymyositis is diagnosed
Both DM and PM are associated with lung, colon, breast, and ovarian cancer.
The risk is approximately 40% for pts > 40 and 66% for male pts > 40.
CXR, colonoscopy, mammogram, and ultrasound are good screening tests.
Occasionally the myositis remits after excision of tumor.

Educate pt on risk of anesthesia
Pts with myopathies are at increased risk for malignant hyperthermia. Careful preoperative evaluation is indicated, and anesthesiologist must be informed of the diagnosis.

Ask about the weakness
Different muscular dystrophies (MD) have different pattern of weakness, muscle group involvement, and time of onset.
Ask about cranial muscle symptoms with droopy eyelids, difficulty chewing, speaking, dysphagia, voice change, and drooling.
Symptoms of proximal muscle weakness include difficulty arising from chair, climbing stairs, reaching higher objects.
Symptoms of distal muscle weakness include dropping things, difficulty opening cans or bottles, hand clumsiness.

Obtain a detailed family history
MD by definition is hereditary. Detailed family history is required.

Are there symptoms of other organ involvement?
MD can affect muscles from other organs. Cardiac muscles are involved frequently. Ask about palpitation, exercise intolerance, and chest pain.
Diaphragm can be affected. Ask about shortness of breath, coughing, and frequent upper respiratory infections.
Weakness affecting smooth muscle of the GI tract will cause constipation.
Some MDs can affect the eyes. Ask about change in vision.
Many pts with MD are mentally retarded.

Perform general physical exam
Auscultate heart for arrhythmia and evidence of cardiomyopathy.
Lens opacity, frontal baldness, and testicular atrophy are suggestive of myotonic dystrophy.

Perform motor exam
Palpate muscle for atrophy. Assess tone and contracture.
Note the pattern of weakness: proximal vs. distal, extensor vs. flexor.
Check for myotonia—ask pt to squeeze your fingers tightly and then let go. Myotonic dystrophy pt will not be able to relax the fists immediately after maximum contraction.
Weakness of paravertebral muscles causes scoliosis, common in Duchenne.
Gower's sign is seen in Duchenne (child attempt to get up from ground with both hands and feet on the floor and works his way up the legs with his hands until in upright posture).
Pseudohypertrophy of calf muscles is seen in Duchenne and Becker. The calf muscle is hypertrophied in response to hip and knee weakness but in fact it is weaker than appeared due to the disease (hence the prefix pseudo).
Gluteus muscle weakness will cause gait to be waddling.
Exaggerated lordosis is caused by weakness of hip extensors.
Standing with feet wide apart (to increase base of support) indicates hip and knee extensor weakness.

Order EMG nerve conduction studies
Will confirm diagnosis in most cases.

Consider muscle biopsy and DNA/chromosome analysis
Muscle biopsy is the gold standard in establishing the diagnosis.
DNA/chromosome analysis will identify the defective gene.

Muscular dystrophies
Inherited disorders manifest as progressive muscle wasting and weakness.
Following are the most common types of MDs listed in order of frequency:
- **Myotonic dystrophy:** Autosomal dominant. Gene is located in chromosome 19q and encodes myotonin protein kinase. Mutation is by *trinucleotide repeat*, which has genetic anticipation. Onset is usually early adulthood, distal hand and facial muscles are affected first and progresses proximally. Cardiac abnormalities are common. Nonmuscular tissues are involved as well—lens opacities, mental retardation, frontal alopecia, testicular atrophy.
- **Duchenne:** X-linked recessive, although 30% cases are sporadic without family history. It is caused by defect in dystrophin gene, which encodes the protein important to muscular structure. Onset is 3 to 6 years of age. Death occurs in late adolescence or 20s. It affects mainly proximal muscles (shoulders and hips).
- **Facioscapulohumeral muscular dystrophy:** Autosomal dominant. Exact gene defect unknown but involves partial deletion of chromosome 4. Onset between 6 and 20 yrs of age. Shoulder and facial muscles are involved. Normal life expectancy.
- **Becker:** It is similar to Duchenne but milder. It is X-linked and involves the same dystrophin gene. Onset is later in teens. Life expectancy is in the 50s.
- **Limb-girdle muscular dystrophies:** A group of MDs characterized by weakness/atrophy in pelvic and shoulder girdles. Face is spared. There are at least 11 subtypes with different gene defect and mode of inheritance.
- **Oculopharyngeal muscular dystrophy:** Autosomal dominant. Gene defect unknown but has been mapped to chromosome 14q. More common in French Canadians and Spanish Americans. Onset after age 45 and main symptoms are bilateral ptosis and dysphagia.
- **Distal muscular dystrophies:** A group of MDs characterized by weakness/atrophy in the distal hand and foot muscles. There are at least four subtypes with different gene defect and mode of inheritance. The onset is in adult life and is more common in those of Swedish descent.
- **Congenital muscular dystrophy:** Autosomal recessive. Onset is at birth or early infancy and characterized by hypotonia and generalized weakness with or without joint contracture. The defect is either in merosin (an extracellular muscle protein) gene on chromosome 6 or its receptor protein (integrin α 7).
- **Emery-Dreifuss muscular dystrophy:** X-linked recessive with defect in gene encoding emerin, a nuclear protein. Onset in late childhood to adulthood. Pt has weakness and contractures in upper arms and proximal and distal legs.

 Supportive care
There is no cure for MDs. Treatment is symptomatic and supportive.
Dilantin and quinine may reduce myotonia.
Maintain a well-balanced diet with adequate fibers or stool softener to prevent constipation.
Weight control. Overweight adds burden to supporting muscles.
Avoid prolonged bed rest, which can accelerate weakening of muscles.
Moderate exercises such as swimming are beneficial.
Passive range of motion exercise will prevent muscle contractures.
Splints or orthotics ± corrective surgeries may prolong ambulation.
MD pts have higher risk of malignant hyperthermia to general anesthesia such as halothane. Anesthesiologist must be notified the diagnosis before surgery.
Respiratory care with chest massage and tracheostomy to prevent pneumonia.
 Genetic counseling and prenatal testing.

S ### Does the pt have any motor symptoms?
Motor symptoms usually start distally in one extremity. Pt may complain of clumsiness in hand, wrist drop, or foot drop.
The symptoms then progress proximally and affect other parts of body. Neck extensors are affected more than flexors.
Pt may experience frequent nocturnal cramps.
Pts may also observe muscle wasting and atrophy.

Does the pt have any bulbar (cranial nerve) signs?
Amyotrophic lateral sclerosis (ALS) may affect the lower cranial motor neurons causing dysarthria, dysphagia, and choking. Weight loss is very common as the result of decreased PO intake.

Does the pt have any respiratory signs?
Dyspnea on exertion and shortness of breath at rest are bad prognostic factors.

Is there a family history of ALS?
10% of ALS cases are hereditary. Inheritance is autosomal dominant. Approximately 20% of these pts have a mutation in superoxide dismutase 1 enzyme (SOD1), which functions as an antioxidant.

Ask about symptoms of cervical cord disease
Clinical picture of ALS is very similar to that of upper spinal cord disease. Ask about bladder/bowel incontinence, any pain in the neck, history of neck trauma.

O ### Perform general physical examination
Assess the general medical condition of the pt. Is the pt cachectic?
Look for signs of conditions that might cause or mimic ALS: hyperthyroidism and hypothyroidism, cancer, autoimmune disorders, and heavy metal poisoning.

Assess the mental status
ALS does not affect the brain. Mental status should be normal at the time of diagnosis when general health is not greatly impaired. Cognitive abnormalities as seen in Alzheimer's disease are not consistent with ALS.
Emotional lability may be seen as part of pseudobulbar effect. Pt may have episode of uncontrollable laughing and/or crying that may be inappropriate or unrelated to the situation at hand.

Check cranial nerves
Extraocular muscles should be full. ALS does not affect ocular muscles.
Speech may be dysarthric.
Voice can have nasal quality.
Look for fasciculation of the tongue in relaxed state.
Gag and jaw-jerk reflexes may be overactive.

Perform detailed motor exam
Hallmark of ALS is presence of *both* upper and lower motor neuron signs.

Upper motor neuron signs: hyperreflexia, ↑ tone or spasticity, and positive Babinski.
Lower motor neuron signs: muscle atrophy and fasciculation. Fasciculation is most easily seen in tongue and big muscles such as thigh and calf muscles.
Presence of parkinsonian features is not consistent with ALS (see chapter on Parkinson) unless the pt is from Guam, where they may have a disease called PD-ALS-Dementia Complex of Guam.

Check anal sphincter tone if no overwhelming findings of ALS
Presence of sphincter tone abnormality is not consistent with ALS. Consider spinal cord disease.

Perform sensory exam
ALS does not affect sensory nerves. If abnormal, consider other diagnosis.

Order EMG/nerve conduction studies (NCS)
EMG/NCS are the gold standard tests in diagnosing ALS.

NCS is necessary to ensure that sensory fibers are spared and no demyelinating features (i.e., conduction block) that may suggest a different diagnosis such as multifocal motor neuropathy.

EMG will show both acute and chronic denervation in muscles.

At least two muscles of different nerves and roots in three of the four body regions (i.e., cervical, lumbar, thoracic, and bulbar) have to be involved to diagnose ALS.

Consider MRI of C-spine and brain
Order only if other diagnosis is suspected (see below).

For ALS, MRI may show increased signal along the corticospinal tract pathways (anterior spinal cord, ventral brainstem, and posterior limb of internal capsule) due to degeneration of upper motor neurons.

Amyotrophic lateral sclerosis
The most common motor neuron disease, affects approximately five per 100,000 people. Onset usually between 40 and 60 years of age. Males affected slightly > females.

ALS involves the anterior horn cells (motor neurons) in the spinal cord and cranial motor neurons in the brainstem. The nerve cells undergo degeneration and cell death. The cause is unknown. The discovery of SOD1 gene (see above) in familial ALS has suggested that oxidative stress, mitochondrial dysfunction, and excitotoxicity pathways may be involved in the process of neuronal cell death.

Carefully consider DDx since many are treatable conditions.
- Other motor neuron diseases: monomelic amyotrophy, adult-onset progressive spinal muscular atrophy, and motor neuronopathies due to paraneoplastic syndrome, irradiation, infections (polio), toxic/heavy-metal, and electrocution.
- Peripheral neuropathies: chronic inflammatory demyelinating polyradioneuropathy, multifocal motor neuropathy
- Cervical myelopathy: cord compression from spondylosis and tumor. Syringomyelia.
- Brain/brainstem disease: syringobulbia, foramen magnum lesions such as meningioma, Arnold-Chiari malformation, prominent white matter disease (e.g., severe chronic small vessel disease, multiple sclerosis, Tay-Sachs disease).

Start riluzole 50 mg PO Q 12 hrs
It is the only FDA-approved medication available to treat ALS. Mechanism of action is not known. It prolongs tracheostomy-free survival period.

Provide prognosis, counseling, and supportive care
Average survival after diagnosis is 5 years. Counseling and support groups may be helpful.

Physical therapy and anti-spasticity and spasm medications (see chapter on spasticity) will provide some relieve.

Pt will eventually need a tracheostomy and G-tube.

S **Does the pt have any pain, numbness, and weakness?**
Depending on the type of nerve involved (motor, sensory, mixed), pt may have weakness and/or sensory changes in the area supplied by the affected nerve.
Ask about the PQRST of the pain (see neuropathic pain chapter).

Ask about the risk factors for developing entrapment neuropathies
Ask about occupation and sports activities. Repetitive use of the wrist, elbow, knee, and ankle causes scarring of soft tissues surrounding the nerve and compresses the already tight space.
Pts with diabetes, rheumatoid arthritis, hypothyroidism, pregnancy, amyloidosis, and acromegaly have higher chance of developing nerve entrapment. It is because of less healthy nerves, soft tissue swelling, and bone expansion.

O **Carefully assess the sensory and motor function in the limb(s) affected**
Nerve entrapment is a focal process. If abnormalities are found outside of the distribution of affected nerve, consider other diagnosis such as plexopathy, radiculopathy, or generalized peripheral neuropathy. Some entrapment syndromes (e.g., carpal tunnel) can be bilateral.
Provocative test is done by forced flexion of the joint with attempt to reproduce symptom (e.g., *Phalen test* for carpal tunnel syndrome, elbow flexion for cubital tunnel syndrome).
Tinel test is done by tapping the affected nerve at the suspected compression site. It is positive if symptom is reproduced (e.g., tapping at the wrist flexor retinaculum for carpal tunnel syndrome [CTS] and tapping the posterior medial maleolus for tarsal tunnel syndrome).
Thumb is a useful finger to assess for injuries of radial (abduction), median (opposition), and ulnar (adduction) nerves.
Look for atrophy in the muscle supplied by the suspected nerve.
Check the sensory over the area supplied by the suspected nerve.
Palpate and examine for any tumor, ganglion cyst, and lipoma in the suspected areas.

Order EMG/nerve conduction studies (NCS)
These are the most important diagnostic tests in nerve entrapment syndromes. They can help localize the lesion, assess the severity of the injury, and at the same time rule out other causes of pt's symptoms (e.g., radiculopathy, plexopathy).
Serial tests may be needed to monitor the progression of injury or response to treatment.

Consider imaging study
MRI is the imaging study of choice because it displays the soft tissues (nerve, muscle, tendons) wells. It also can detect tumors such as lipomas and ganglions, as well as aneurysms and rheumatoid synovitis.
X-ray study if fracture is suspected.

Common nerve entrapment syndromes: carpal tunnel syndrome
CTS is the most common entrapment neuropathy. It is caused by the compression of median nerve as it goes through the carpal tunnel at the wrist.
Pt presents with numbness, tingling, and neuropathic type of pain in the hand extending up to the forearm and elbow. The symptom is usually worse at night.
Occupations at risk for developing CTS include factory assemblers, typists, secretaries, musicians, and programmers. The use of highly repetitive wrist movements, vibrating tools, awkward wrist positions, and great force seems to be correlated with the disorder. Pregnancy is also associated with CTS.

Ulnar neuropathies

The ulnar nerve is most commonly being compressed in the cubital tunnel at the elbow followed by Guyon canal at the wrist.

Ulnar neuropathy at the elbow can occur with elbow fracture, subluxation, external compression, and overuse of the elbow with scarring of the aponeurosis and ligaments.

At the wrist, the Guyon canal can be narrowed by ganglion, tumor, or repetitive use.

Pt complains of numbness and in the fourth, fifth finger, medial side of hand, and forearm.

Wrist drop

Caused by damage to the radial or posterior interosseous nerve (deep motor branch of the radial nerve coming off supinator).

Causes include dislocations of the elbow, fractures, rheumatoid arthritis, soft tissue tumors, ganglia and traumatic or developmental fibrous bands.

Damage to posterior interosseous nerve causes weakness of the digital extensors (finger drop). No sensory symptoms. This is different from radial nerve palsy (wrist drop) which causes numbness in the dorsum of hand.

Foot drop (peroneal neuropathy)

Caused by damage to the deep peroneal nerve or the common peroneal nerve. The most common cause is compression at the fibular head. It's a common post-op complication.

Pure deep peroneal nerve injury will cause dorsiflexion weakness and numbness in first dorsal web space. If foot eversion is also weak then the common peroneal nerve is involved. If knee flexion is weak too that means the sciatic or L5 nerve root is involved.

Meralgia paresthetica

Caused by compression of the pure sensory lateral femoral cutaneous nerve (LFCN). Usually seen in obese individuals or women in third trimester of pregnancy. The heavy abdomen pushes the inguinal ligament forward and downward and at the same time drags and stretches LFCN.

The sensory deficit is on the lateral thighs (similar to areas covered by pants side pockets).

The symptoms are usually worse with walking down slopes or stairs, prolonged standing, and lying flat. Symptoms are relieved by placing a pillow behind the thighs and assuming a slightly hunched posture while standing.

Tarsal tunnel syndrome

Caused by the compression of tibial nerve as it passes through the tarsal tunnel underneath flexor retinaculum in the medial ankle.

Seen in pts with flat feet, diabetes, cyst, rheumatoid arthritis, ankle fractures, or repetitive use.

Pt presents with numbness, pain, and burning in the ankle, heel, and sole of the foot.

Attempt medical treatment

NSAIDs are good for anti-inflammatory and pain control.

Wrist splints, ankle support, or orthotics to keep the affected joint in neutral position for day and night use.

Steroid injection at the affected sites. PO steroid may be helpful as well.

Consider surgical treatment

Surgery is indicated if pt fails medical therapy or if EMG/NCS shows severe neuropathy with axonal loss.

S Is there weakness on one side of the face?
Most pts with Bell's palsy present to the emergency department (ED) thinking they had a stroke. Often diagnosis is not clear to the ED physician who then consults a neurologist.
Pt will often complain their face is pulled to one side. The side of pulling is actually the healthy side.
Drooling is also common and is on the same side of the lesion.

Was there pain behind the ear?
Pain behind the ear on the affected side 1 to 2 days before the attack is a very common symptom.

Is there change in taste?
This is also a common symptom and indicates the lesion is at or proximal to the point where chorda tympani fibers join the facial nerve.

Is there change in hearing?
Hyperacusis is due to paralysis of the stapedius muscle, which is supplied by the facial nerve.

Is there numbness in the face?
The sensory loss can be in one or two distribution of trigeminal nerve. It is unclear why numbness occurs but it is not uncommon.

Are there risk factors for Bell's palsy?
Pregnancy (especially third trimester), diabetes, thyroid disease, and immunocompromised state are the most common conditions; however, most of the time there is no association with any underlying conditions.

Are there any other focal neurologic symptoms?
Such as hemiparesis, hemisensory loss, double vision. If yes, then it's more likely to be a stroke than Bell's palsy.

Examine the face carefully
Watch the face at rest and note any asymmetry. The palpebral fissure on the affected side is larger due to weakness of orbicularis oculi.
Ask pt to smile or show teeth. Observe for any asymmetry.
Ask pt to wrinkle forehead, which should be asymmetric as well. If it is symmetric, then pt may have stroke although sometimes the asymmetry is very subtle and difficult to tell.
Use a cotton tip to do corneal reflex. Note symmetry in the blinking response (facial nerve supplies orbicularis oculi which closes the eyes). The affected side will blink slower.

Examine the ears and hearing
Checking hearing. The affected side may exhibit hyperacusis.
Examine the external auditory canal for vesicles that indicate Ramsay-Hunt syndrome, which is due to infection of the geniculate ganglion by herpes zoster virus.
Examine the tympanic membrane. Complicated OM can cause facial palsy.

Check taste
Facial nerve supplies the anterior two thirds of the tongue. Use a cotton swab and test the sides of tongue with any sweet things you can find (e.g., soda, orange juice). Ask pt to close eyes and see if he/she is able to taste on both good side and bad side.

Finish the rest of neurologic exam
If any focality, then pt has stroke and not Bell's palsy.

Send laboratory studies
Routine labs should include electrolytes, glucose, CBC, rapid plasma reagin, thyroid-stimulating hormone
If facial palsy is recurrent or bilateral, send HIV, ACE, and Lyme titer.

Consider EMG/nerve conduction studies (NCS)
These tests are used to assess the function of facial nerve and are used mainly for prognosis. This is not part of acute workup.

Bell's palsy
Fairly common with incidence of 23 per 100,000 annually. Affects all age groups, both genders equally, and throughout the year.

The exact cause is unknown but is speculated to be due to herpes simplex virus infection. The nerve goes through the tight facial canal in temporal bone. As the nerve gets inflamed and swollen, it is prone to get compressed, infarcted, and demyelinated.

The differential diagnosis includes stroke in the pons, parotid tumors, acoustic neuroma, basilar artery aneurysm, syphilis, Lyme, HIV, and Ramsay-Hunt syndrome (varicella zoster virus).

It is uncommon for Bell's palsy to recur (approximately 8%). It is even rarer for facial palsy to be bilateral, especially simultaneously. When this is the case, other causes of CN7 palsy should be ruled out: Guillain-Barré syndrome, Lyme disease, HIV, sarcoidosis, Möbius syndrome, and Melkersson-Rosenthal syndrome.

Prescribe antiviral medication
Controversial whether it is beneficial, but it is standard practice.
Acyclovir 800 mg PO five times per day for 7 days.

Start corticosteroids
Steroids may help decrease swelling especially in the tight facial canal.
Prednisone 60 mg PO QD for 7 days followed by quick taper.

Educate about eye care
The lacrimal gland is innervated by the greater petrosal nerve, which is a branch of the facial nerve. Also, weakness of orbicularis oculi will cause difficulty closing the eye. The cornea may be susceptible to drying and foreign body exposure.
Use artificial tears PRN.
Tape the eye shut when sleeping at night. Alternatively use lubricant before going to bed.
Eyeglasses or shield to protect against foreign objects and minimize airflow to the cornea.

Prognosis
Pts are often anxious about the cosmetic effect of Bell's palsy.
Approximately 80% of pts have complete recovery within a few weeks.
Early recovery of some motor function in the first 5 to 7 days is the most favorable prognostic sign.
If symptom does not get better after 10 days, there is likely Wallerian degeneration present. Obtain EMG/NCS; if there is evidence of denervation, the recovery may take a long time (months to years).
When the nerves regenerate, the fibers may misroute and innervate adjacent tissues. Examples include *synkinesis* (when eye blinks the corner of mouth will twitch) and "crocodile tears" (tearing when eating, caused by misrouting of greater petrosal nerve fibers with chorda tympani).

IX
Neuro-Oncology

Is the pt experiencing any symptoms of brain tumors?
For tumors in the cerebral hemisphere, seizures are the most common presentation.
For tumors in the posterior fossa: ataxia and cranial nerve signs.
For spinal cord: paraparesis, sensory loss, and urinary incontinence.
If the tumor arises within the ventricles or near the cerebral aqueduct, pt may present with symptoms of ↑ intracranial pressure (ICP), such as headache, nausea, vomiting.

What is the age group?
Age is the most important clue to generate a differential diagnosis of tumor type.

Perform a general physical exam
The most common brain tumor is metastasis. Look for signs of malignancy, which include cachexia, lymphadempathy, asymmetric breath sound, breast mass, skin lesions.

Perform complete neurologic exam
Signs of tumor are often subtle relative to the size and extent of the lesion.
Assess for signs of increased ICP.
Assess cortical function: speech, visual-spatial, visual fields, neglect, memory.
Assess cranial nerves, including visual acuity (for optic glioma).
Look for subtle motor and reflex asymmetry. Check Babinski response.

Obtain image of the brain with and without contrast
MR spectroscopy may aide in determining tumor versus non-tumor lesions.

Common brain tumors
Astrocytoma: originates from astrocyte (the main glial supporting cell in the CNS).
- Can be divided into two major categories, diffuse and circumscribed. Diffused astrocytoma cannot be resected completely while circumscribed astrocytoma can (therefore better prognosis).
- Diffused astrocytoma is graded by the World Health Organization. Grade I is low grade with average survival of 7 years while grade IV (glioblastoma multiforme) has average survival of 1 year.
- Circumscribed astrocytoma include pilocytic astrocytoma (second most common pediatric brain tumor), pleomorphic xanthoastrocytomas, and subependymal giant cell astrocytoma (common in tuberous sclerosis).

Ependymoma: originates from ependymal cells (lining of ventricles and central canal).
- Occurs in all ages, but more common in children (third most common).
- The most common cerebral site is within the fourth ventricle. Patients often present with hydrocephalus and increased ICP.
- Perivascular rosettes are the pathology hallmark.
- Myxopapillary ependymoma is a subtype that is exclusively found in cauda equina and conus medullaris. More common in adults and pts present with cauda equina syndrome.
- Prognosis varies widely. Survival ranges from < 1 yr to > 10 yrs.

Oligodendroglioma: originates from oligodendrocyte (produces myelin sheath in CNS).
- "Fried egg" appearance under microscope is the hallmark. On CT scan they often have calcification and hemorrhage.
- Median survival is 8 yrs for low-grade and 3 yrs for high-grade.

Primitive neuroectodermal tumors (PNET): consist of cells that resemble neuroectodermal precursors (embryologically, neuroectoderm gives rise to neural plate and neural groove, which spawn neurons, glial cells, adrenal medulla, dura, melanocytes).
- PNET of CNS include medulloblastoma, neuroblastoma, and pineoblastoma. PNET of non-CNS include adrenal neuroblastoma and retinoblastoma. Homer

Wright rosettes are the pathologic hallmark.
- Medulloblastoma is the most common pediatric brain tumor. Occurs in children < 10 y/o and less commonly 18 to 25 y/o. Originates in midline cerebellum, is highly malignant, and will metastasize along CSF pathways. Surgery followed by radiation to entire neuraxis and chemotherapy are standard treatment with mean survival of 10 years.

Meningioma: arises from arachnoid cells in the arachnoid.
- Common in people > 50 y/o but are seen in children as well. More common in females probably due to presence of progesterone and estrogen receptors on the tumor. Most are associated with abnormalities on chromosome 22. Pts with NF2 often have multiple meningiomas.
- Most common locations, in descending order of frequency, are cerebral convexity, parasagittal region, sphenoid wing, parasellar region, and spinal canal. Clinical presentation depends on the location of tumor.
- They have tendency to encircle on another, forming calcified whorls called *psammoma bodies*, which are the hallmark of meningiomas.

Malformative tumors and cysts: originate from embryonal cell rests within CNS.
- Craniopharyngioma grows from epithelial rests derived from Rathke's pouch, which is the embryonic precursor of adenophysis. It is located in the intrasellar or suprasellar location and often encroaches on the third ventricle causing hydrocephalus.
- Lipoma tends to occur at midline structures: corpus callosum, midbrain, cerebellar vermis, and spinal cord. Seizures are caused by mass effect.
- Colloid cyst is a ball-like structure formed by a lining of epithelial cells with mucinous material inside. Located in third ventricle and may produce positional hydrocephalus due to "ball-valve" effect at the foramen of Monro.
- Epidermoid (pearly tumor) and dermoid cysts are formed by epithelial cells that contain keratin (epidermoid) or skin adnexae (dermoid). They can arise anywhere in CNS. Leakage of the cyst contents can cause chemical meningitis.

Metastatic tumors: in order of frequency: lung, breast, melanoma, renal, GI tumors. They tend to metastasize to gray-white matter junction in middle cerebral artery territory. Prostate, cervical, sarcomas, and squamous cell carcinoma almost never metastasize to brain.

P Address acute issues first
Start corticosteroid to decrease the mass effect and surrounding edema.
Load and start phenytoin if pt has seizure.
Insert ventriculoperitoneal shunt or other measures if increased ICP.

Obtain tissue sample
Biopsy is the gold standard to establishing tumor diagnosis and grade. Consult neurosurgery. Available options are stereotactic biopsy and open surgery. Rapid frozen section during surgery will give surgeon immediate guide as how to approach the tumor.

Consult radiation oncology and neuro-oncology
Dealing with brain tumor is a complicated issue and a multidisciplinary approach is recommended.

S **Does the pt have any visual symptoms?**
The optic chiasm lies approximately 1 cm above the pituitary fossa and is susceptible to compression from pituitary mass.
Common visual complaints include progressive loss of central acuity and dimming of the visual field, especially in its temporal portion.
Diplopia can occur if the mass expands laterally to compress the cavernous sinus affecting CN3, CN4, and CN6.

Does the pt have nasal symptoms?
The pituitary fossa lies above the sphenoid sinus and nasal septum and may cause sinusitis, epistaxis, nasal obstruction, and CSF leak.

Does the pt have headache?
The mass can expand upward and obstruct the third ventricle, causing hydrocephalus. Even without hydrocephalus, pituitary tumor alone can cause headache, which is often described as bitemporal or periorbital.

Does the pt have symptoms of endocrinopathy?
Both hypopituitarism and hyperpituitarism are possible, although hyperpituitarism is more common. Prolactin, growth hormone, adrenocortical hormone, and thyroid-stimulating hormone are the hormones secreted by anterior pituitary. Antidiuretic hormone and oxytocin are produced by the posterior pituitary.
- Hyperprolactinemia: infertility, amenorrhea, galactorrhea, gonadal dysfunction
- Acromegaly: gigantism, diabetes mellitus (DM), entrapment neuropathies
- Cushing's: amenorrhea, impotence, DM, central obesity, acne, muscle wasting
- Hyperthyroidism: fatigue, weight loss, palpitation, heat intolerance, diarrhea
- Diabetes insipidus: excessive thirst and frequent urination

 Assess vital signs
Hypertension is frequently seen in hyperprolactinemia, acromegaly, and Cushing's disease.
Hyperthermia and hypothermia can be a sign of hypothalamic dysfunction.

Perform general exam
Look for signs of the endocrinopathies listed above.

Carefully test visual acuity and fields
The classic visual field defect is *bitemporal homonymous hemianopsia*; however, there may be a variety of other visual field cuts.
Visual acuity and color perception may be affected in one or both eyes.
Check extraocular muscles for CN3, CN4, or CN6 palsy.

Send laboratory studies
Prolactin level should be checked in all cases. The other hormone levels can be ordered based on clinical suspicion.
"Stalk section effect" is a phenomenon in which a non–prolactin-secreting mass causes elevation in prolactin level by compressing the pituitary stalk. The hypothalamus secretes dopamine and other prolactin-inhibiting factors that suppress the pituitary release of prolactin. By compressing the stalk, there is loss of inhibition, which results in elevated prolactin release.
Prolactin level < 2500 mU/L is suggestive of stalk section effect, while level > 2500 mU/L is more consistent with prolactinoma.
Dynamic hormone tests can be performed to assess the functionality of the tumor. These tests include dexamethasone suppression test, thyroid releasing hormone, growth hormone–releasing hormone, corticotropin-releasing hormone, metyrapone,

gonadotropin-releasing hormone tests. Consult endocrinology to assist in performing these tests.

Obtain MRI of brain and sella with and without contrast
MRI is the test of choice and establishes the diagnosis most of the time.

Pituitary tumors
Tumors in the pituitary region can arise either from the pituitary itself or from non-pituitary origin. Tumors from the anterior pituitary (adenohypophysis) include adenoma and carcinoma. Tumors from the posterior pituitary (neurohypophysis) include granular cell tumor and astrocytoma.

Non-pituitary origin tumors in the sella include craniopharyngioma, germ cell tumor, glioma, meningioma, chordoma, lipoma, chondroma, sarcoma, schwannoma, metastasis.

Other non-neoplastic causes of pituitary mass include Rathke's cyst, empty sella syndrome, pituitary apoplexy, sarcoidosis, internal carotid artery aneurysm, cavernous malformation, lymphocytic hypophysitis, and giant cell granuloma.

Pituitary adenoma is the most common cause of pituitary gland lesion.

Pituitary adenoma is very common. It's found in approximately 20% of population at postmortem; the majority were asymptomatic.

Pituitary adenoma causes symptoms in one of three ways:
- Pituitary hyperfunction due to hormone hypersecretion.
- Pituitary hypofunction due to compression of normal pituitary tissue.
- Mass effect on adjacent tissues (e.g., superiorly optic chiasm and third ventricle, laterally cavernous sinus, inferiorly sphenoid sinus).

Decide whether pt needs treatment
Many times pituitary adenomas are discovered incidentally. If pt is asymptomatic, no treatment is needed and the tumor can be followed with yearly MRI scan.

Initiate medical therapy
For prolactin-secreting adenoma, start bromocriptine at 0.5 mg QD and slowly titrate up until a therapeutic response is obtained. Most of the pts will respond well to bromocriptine with shrinking of tumor and a decrease in prolactin level.

For acromegaly, bromocriptine might work but octreotide (a somatostatin analogue) is preferred choice. Start at 200 mg/day and increase by 200 mg/wk to goal of 1600 mg/day.

Pts will need biannual hormone levels checked and brain MRI.

Consider surgical resection
Surgery is indicated if pt fails or could not tolerate medical therapy.

Approach is transsphenoidal through the nose. Success rate is high if tumor can be completely resected.

Radiation is also a reasonable option or if pt has failed surgery.

X
Pain

S **What is the quality of headache?**
Dull and aching headaches usually arise from structures deep to the skin.
Sharp pain usually indicates pain from superficial structures such as skin and scalp.

Is the headache throbbing or pulsatile?
Throbbing pain usually indicates vascular origin and is characteristic of migraine.

How intense is the pain?
The pain scale 1 to 10 is the most commonly used, but is subjective and yields little information. A better index of severity is the degree to which the pain has incapacitated the patient (e.g., missing school work).

Where is the headache?
Unilateral throbbing headache is very characteristic of migraine.
Pain in the temporal area may be due to temporal arteritis.

How rapid did the headache start?
Subarachnoid hemorrhage headache starts abruptly within seconds.
Tension and migraine headaches start within minutes.
Meningitis and encephalitis headaches develop over several hours to days.
Headaches from intracranial tumor may develop slowly over days to months and waxes and wanes.

Is the headache recurrent and how frequent is the headache?
Recurrent headaches are from migraine, tension, cluster, rebound, and tumor.
Migraine usually occurs once every few weeks.
Tension headache can be as frequent as daily to once every few months.
Cluster headache usually occurs in clusters with nightly attacks for several days to weeks.
Rebound headache from analgesic overuse is almost always daily.

Does the headache wake pt at night?
Intracranial tumors often wakes pt at night.
Cluster headache usually begins 1 or 2 hrs after pt falls asleep.

Does the headache change with supine or prone position?
Because of gravity, intracranial pressure is higher when one is flat and lower when upright.
Headaches from diseases that increase intracranial pressure (ICP) such as brain tumor and pseudotumor cerebri become worse when pt is lying flat.
Headaches from processes that decrease ICP such as post–lumbar puncture and VP shunt become worse when pt stands up.

What makes the headache better and what makes it worse?
Headache from cervical spine is usually worse after periods of inactivity such as a night's sleep.
Brain mass headaches may worsen with straining, coughing, or lifting.
Migraine headache may get worse with bright light and noise and get better when pt goes into dark quiet room.
Sinus headache may become worse with stooping and change in atmospheric pressure. It is also usually worse upon awakening if pt has allergy.

Are there focal neurologic complaints?
If pt has no neurologic complaints (hemiparesis, numbness, visual change, speech and swallowing difficulties, seizures, mental status change) then the headache is more likely to be benign in nature (e.g., tension, migraine, cluster).

Perform a complete general physical and neurologic exam
Fever may indicate meningitis, encephalitis.
Check for neck stiffness for meningitis.
Obese female pt raises suspicion for pseudotumor cerebri.
Perform funduscopic exam to rule of papilledema as seen in pseudotumor cerebri or other disease with elevated ICP.
Auscultate the skull and orbits for bruit as heard with arteriovenous malformations and fistulas.
Arteries may be tender and harden to palpation in temporal arteritis.
Palpate and tap the sinus for tenderness in sinus headache.

Obtain basic screening laboratory studies
Chemistry panel, CBC, urinalysis, liver function tests.
ESR is elevated in temporal arteritis.

Consider brain imaging
Depending on the clinical setting and differential diagnosis, CT or MRI may be indicated.

Consider lumbar puncture
Lumbar puncture should be obtained in suspected subarachnoid hemorrhage (SAH), infections, and pseudotumor cerebri. Check for opening pressure, cell count, glucose, and protein.

Headache
Headache is extremely common and is one of the most common reasons pt seeks medical help. In a given year, approximately 90% of men and 95% of women have had at least one headache.
Within the cranium, the structures that are innervated by trigeminal pain fibers are blood vessels, meninges, and skull. The brain itself is insensitive to pain. Headache occurs when there is meningeal irritation or the presence of pressure and traction on the blood vessels.
Pain is referred to the forehead in anterior cranial fossa lesions; to the face or temple in middle fossa lesions; and to the occiput, neck, and shoulders in posterior fossa lesions.
When evaluating the headache pt for the first time, the physician needs to determine whether the headache is primary or secondary.
1. Primary headaches are benign headaches, meaning there is no underlying organic or structural lesion. Primary headaches include migraine with/without aura, cluster, tension, and rebound headaches. More than 90% of all headaches are primary.
2. Secondary headaches are malignant headaches, meaning there is underlying organic or structural lesion. Some of the common secondary headaches encountered are due to: brain tumor, SAH, temporal arteritis, meningitis, encephalitis. Less than 10% of all headaches are secondary.

Treat the underlying cause, if any
Refer to the notes on SAH, meningitis, tumor.

Treat the headache itself
Refer to the notes on migraine, tension, cluster headache.

Does aura precede the headache?
An aura is a transient disturbance of nervous function. Common migraine auras include (from most to least common):
- Visual changes, which can include blurry vision, photopsia (flashes of light), scotoma (enlarged blind spot), teichopsia (dazzling zigzag lines).
- Sensory disturbances such as numbness of face, lips, and hands.
- Motor disturbances such as weakness or numbness of arms and legs.
- Language disturbances such as aphasia, dysarthria.
- Balance disturbances such as dizziness, vertigo, and unsteady gait.
- Mental status change such as drowsiness and confusion.

Migraine with aura is also known as classic migraine.

Migraine without aura is also known as common migraine, which is five times more common than classic migraine.

What is the headache like?
Migraine headache is most commonly described as (1) unilateral, (2) throbbing, (3) moderate to severe to interfere with daily activity, and (4) aggravated by physical activity.
At least two of the four features are needed for the diagnosis.

Is there associated symptom during the attack?
Nausea, vomiting, photophobia, phonophobia. At least one has to be present for the diagnosis.

What makes the headache better?
Pt usually finds relief by going into dark and quiet room or by sleeping.

How long does the headache last?
Migraine attacks last between 4 and 72 hrs. If the headache lasts longer, then it's unlikely to be migraine or migraine alone.

Is the headache recurrent?
By definition, migraine has to be recurrent. The frequency varies from weeks to months. If pt has migraine every day or every few days then he/she is likely to have tension or rebound headache mixed with migraine.
For migraine with aura, at least two episodes are needed for the diagnosis.
For migraine without aura, at least five episodes are required.

Is there family history of migraine?
Migraine has strong genetic component. Positive family history strongly supports diagnosis of migraine. There is no clear Mendelian inheritance pattern.

Perform a complete general and neurologic exam
Except for minority of pts with migraine variants, all pts with migraine should have a normal neurologic exam. History is the key to the diagnosis.

In pts with complicated migraine, neurologic deficit occurs during the attack and outlasts the headache. The deficit may last days and may be permanent. Etiology is thought to be due to ischemia. Common findings include hemiparesis, numbness, ophthalmoplegia, ataxia, and aphasia.

Migraine headache
Migraine is very common, affecting 6% of men and 18% of women.
The exact pathophysiology is unknown. It may have something to do with dopamine and serotonin receptor in the cerebral blood vessels. There is evidence of both cerebral vascular dilatation and constriction during the migraine.

Start treatment for acute migraine attack
There are a variety of medications for acute migraine headache. Selection depends on the severity of symptoms. Often, it is trial and error.
For mild migraine headache, start with acetaminophen or NSAIDs such as aspirin, ibuprofen, and naproxen.
If no relief from these treatments, use a combination analgesic such as acetaminophen or aspirin plus caffeine.
For moderate to severe migraine, consider the following class of medications:
 1. Triptans: They are serotonin 1B/1D agonists. They are the most effective acute treatment. They include sumatriptan, naratriptan, rizatriptan, zolmitriptan, eletriptan, frovatriptan, and almotriptan. Sumatriptan and zolmitriptan are available as a nasal spray and are indicated in severe migraine.
 2. Ergot alkaloids and derivatives: This class of medication includes ergotamine and dihydroergotamine. There are many formulations: IV, SC, IM, PO, and nasal spray. Choose according to pt preference and clinical setting.
 3. Opioids: They are reserved for rescue therapy when the above medications fail and often are used in the emergency department for refractory migraine. Prescribe with caution.

Guard against rebound headache (medication-overuse headache)
Frequent use of acute medications (simple or mixed analgesic, ergotamine, opiates, and triptans) causes rebound headache.
Try to limit acute therapy to 2 headache days per week on a regular basis. Pts with medication overuse should be given prophylactic treatment (see subsequent section).

Consider migraine prophylaxis therapy
The indications for starting prophylactic therapy include frequent headaches, overuse of acute medications, adverse events with acute therapies, pt preference, and presence of uncommon migraine conditions such as complicated migraine or migraines with prolonged aura.
There are a number of prophylactic medications, the most commonly prescribed are tricyclics, β-blockers, Ca channel blockers, and anti-epileptic medications such as Depakote, Tegretol, and Neurontin.
Injecting botulinum toxin into sensitive temporalis and other cranial muscles can prevent migraine.

Encourage pt to identify and avoid triggers
Common triggers include stress; oral contraceptive drugs; certain foods, such as chocolate, cheese, onions; EtOH, strong odor; changes in barometric pressure; hunger; sleep deprivation; or sudden jarring of head. Prevention is the best migraine treatment.

Ask the pt to describe the headache
Typically tension headache is dull and aching. Other common descriptions include fullness, tightness, and band-like pressure around the head.
Cluster headache is typically described as unilateral, orbital, intense, and nonthrobbing. It often radiates into the forehead, temple, and cheek.

What is the time course of the headache?
Tension headache is usually gradual in onset and may last for days, weeks, months, or even years.
Cluster headache tends to occur nightly 1 to 2 hrs after onset of sleep or several times during the day and night. The headache recurs regularly each day for periods that last over 6 to 12 weeks. The headache then goes away and comes back after many months or years. EtOH precipitates attacks.

Are there any associated symptoms?
Tension headache usually does not have associated symptoms, although many tension headache sufferers are depressed and may exhibit fatigue, anxiety, and depression.
Cluster is associated with blocked nostril, rhinorrhea, injected conjunctivum, lacrimation, miosis, and a flush and edema of the cheek. Some pts will have ptosis on the side of symptom.

What relieves the symptoms?
Tension headache sufferers often report there is nothing that helps the headache. Some of them will report benefit from massage and sleep.
For cluster headache, most pts will arise from bed during an attack and sit in a chair and rock or pace the floor, holding a hand to the side of the head.

Ask about symptoms of depression and anxiety
If pt has chronic headache unresponsive to medical therapy, look into possible psychiatric cause. In my experience, addressing the underlying depression or anxiety disorder often makes the headache go away.

Get detailed history of analgesic usage
Many pts do not consider over-the-counter drugs as medications and will not tell physicians. If pt has chronic headaches and is taking multiple tablets of pain killer daily, then it is very likely pt is experiencing rebound headaches.

 Perform a general physical and neurologic exam
Tension headache pts usually have normal physical exam.
Attention should be paid to rule out secondary headache (see Headache, p. 110).
For cluster headache, there may be associated autonomic signs:
- Ipsilateral nasal congestion
- Rhinorrhea
- Lacrimation
- Injected conjunctiva
- Palpebral edema
- Horner's syndrome

Pts with cluster headache often have the following features:
- Leonine facial appearance
- Thick skin with prominent folds
- Broad chin
- Vertical forehead creases
- Nasal telangiectasia
- Tall stature

Tension Headache
It is extremely common, especially in women.
It tends to start in middle age and coincide with stressful time of life.
The exact mechanism is unclear. One of the hypotheses is that tension headaches are due to excessive contraction of craniocervical muscles and an associated constriction of the scalp arteries.

Cluster Headache
Cluster headache is not that common. Prevalence is estimated to be < 1% of the general population.
It occurs predominantly in young adult men (range 20 to 50 yrs) with male-to-female ratio about 5:1.
Paroxysmal hemicrania is a headache disorder similar to cluster headache. Pts respond very well to indomethacin.

Treat the tension headache
Start out with NSAIDs or acetaminophen.
If simple analgesics are not effective, can try combination analgesics with caffeine and barbiturates.
In general, narcotics should be avoided.
Will also need to address the concurrent depression and anxiety disorder, if any.
Regular exercise, stretching, balanced meals, and adequate sleep should also be part of the headache treatment plan.

Treat cluster headache
If the attack occurs regularly at night. Have pt take ergotamine 2 mg PO before going to bed. It may prevent the headache from occurring.
Once the headache has started, inhalation of 100% oxygen for 10 to 15 minutes at the onset of headache may also abort the attack.
If oxygen is not available, can consider using one of the triptans (see Migraine, p. 112) for abortive therapy as well.
For prophylaxis, verapamil up to 480 mg/day can be used. Lithium is also effective.
Some people will give a short course of corticosteroid over few days to abolish the cluster of headache.

If rebound headache is an issue
Tell the pt the cause of his/her daily headaches and the importance of their coming off these medications.
Taper off the over-the-counter pain killers slowly over weeks.
If necessary start a long-acting pain med such as methadone. Because it is long acting, pt does not experience rebound or withdrawal phase.
Eventually pt will need to be tapered off long-acting pain medications.

116 Neuropathic Pain

S **Ask about the pain and any abnormal sensations**
Inquire about PQRST of the pain
- Provocation and palliation
  - Neuropathic pain often is provoked by everyday innocuous environmental stimuli (allodynia) such as gentle touch, pressure of clothing, wind, and hot/cold temperature.
  - Hyperalgesia is exaggerated pain sensation in response to normal painful stimuli.
- Quality and quantity
  - Pain is often described as deep aching, burning, lancinating, or electric shock-like.
  - There may be abnormal sensations such as paresthesia (altered sensitivity to touch), hyperesthesia (exaggerated response to touch), and dysesthesia (painful to touch).
- Region and radiation
  - Ask about the distribution of the pain and radiation. Shooting pain from back or neck is suggestive of radiculopathy. Shooting pain from wrist to fingers or elbow is suggestive of carpal tunnel syndrome.
- Severity and scale
  - Rate the pain from scale of 1 (no pain) to 10 (worst pain).
  - How does the pain affect pt's life and everyday activities?
- Timing and type of onset
  - Neuropathic pain can be constant and/or intermittent. Pt may have constant burning sensation in the feet with intermittent electric-shock pain.

Does pt have conditions that cause neuropathic pain?
Causes of neuropathic pain are listed subsequently. Ask about history of diabetes, EtOH use, HIV risk factors, herpes zoster, strokes, cancer, and drug history.

 Perform general physical exam
The goal of general physical is to assess non-neurologic cause of pain such as musculoskeletal, inflammatory, myofascial, and psychological.
Check for ↓ range of motion, joint stiffness, localized tenderness, and trigger points.

Perform neurologic exam
Localize where the nerve damage (central vs. peripheral, root vs. plexus vs. individual nerves, diffuse vs. localized).
Refer to the chapter on peripheral neuropathy.
Allodynia (pain in response to a innocuous stimuli) and hyperalgesia (increased pain in response to a normally painful stimuli) are frequently seen.

Consider ancillary studies
Only if the cause of neuropathic pain is unclear. If central cause is suspected, consider imaging of the spine or brain. If peripheral, consider EMG/nerve conduction studies (NCS) and other tests to establish the cause.

 Neuropathic pain
Very common. Prevalence of people with neuropathic pain is unknown. For painful diabetic neuropathy alone, there are more than 3 million sufferers. Incidence of neuropathic pain goes up with age.
The underlying pathophysiology of neuropathic pain is poorly understood. The process of generation of neuropathic pain is thought to involve (1) increased afferent nociceptor firing, (2) decreased inhibition of neuronal activity in central structure, and (3) altered central processing so that normal sensory input is amplified and sustained.

Both central and peripheral nervous lesion can cause neuropathic pain.
Peripheral causes include:
- Diabetes
- CIDP
- Reflex sympathetic dystrophy
- Radiculopathy
- Trigeminal neuralgia
- Postherpetic neuralgia
- Heavy metal poisoning
- Postsurgical
- EtOH
- Drugs (chemo, INH, B6)
- Nerve entrapment (e.g., carpal tunnel)
- Post-traumatic
- Post-radiation
- Phantom limb
- HIV sensory neuropathy
- Nutritional deficiency (e.g., vitamin B_{12})

Central causes of neuropathic pain include:
- Stroke
- Parkinson disease
- Compressive myelopathy
- Posttraumatic spinal cord injury
- Multiple sclerosis
- HIV myelopathy
- Postradiation myelopathy
- Syringomyelia

Correct or treat the underlying cause
If the identified cause is correctable (e.g., carpal tunnel) or treatable (e.g., diabetes mellitus), the primary effort should be to optimize the control of disease.

Symptomatic pain control
There are a variety of medications that works for neuropathic pain. Treatment should be individualized, taking into account the side-effect profile, type of pain, severity, distribution of pain, and pt's age. The following are the most commonly prescribed neuropathic pain medications:
- Gabapentin: Start at 100 mg PO TID and titrate up by 100 mg Q 3 days to 1800 mg/day or when symptom is controlled. If total dose required is > 3600 mg/day, then the dose should be divided QID because gabapentin does not get well absorbed at dose > 1200 mg. Most common side effect is sedation.
- Duloxetine: A serotonin and norepinephrine reuptake inhibitor antidepressant recently approved by FDA for treatment of painful diabetic neuropathy. Start at 30 mg PO QD and titrate up to120 mg/day.
- Amitryptyline, nortriptyline or desipramine: Start at 25 mg PO QHS, and titrate up by 25 mg Q 7 days up to 150 mg QHS. Be careful in elderly with cardiac disease, glaucoma, and urinary retention. They may be beneficial in pts with depression because they are antidepressants as well.
- Carbamazepine: The first-line agent for trigeminal neuralgia. Start 200 mg BID and titrate up until symptom is controlled.
- Tramadol: A norepinephrine and serotonin reuptake inhibitor with opioid agonist activity. It may be beneficial in pts with concurrent musculoskeletal or arthritic pain. Start at 50 mg PO QD and titrate up by 50 mg Q 7 days to 100 mg QID.
- 5% Lidocaine patch: Apply TID to the painful area. Systemic drug level is minimal and therefore there is no side effect except possible local skin irritation. It may be helpful in elderly with multiple medical problems on numerous medications.
- Opioid analgesics: Usually reserved as last-line given its side effects and abuse potential. Start with short-acting ones such as oxycodone or hydrocodone for 1 to 2 wks and then convert to equi-analgesic daily dosage of the long-acting ones such as methadone, levorphanol, fentanyl patch, or controlled-release morphine.

XI
Neuro-Immunology

Does the pt have any of the four common presentations of multiple sclerosis (MS)?
Optic neuritis (monocular blurry vision, blindness).
Transverse myelitis (paraparesis, bladder incontinence/retention).
Brainstem signs (diplopia, dysphagia, dysarthria).
Cerebellar ataxia (vertigo, unsteadiness).

What is the age and gender of the pt?
MS is a disease of young people. Two thirds of cases have their onset between 20 and 40 years of age. Majority of the rest had their first symptom started before age 20.
Incidence of MS is two to three times higher in women than men.
Young female pt presenting with focal neurologic symptom, it's MS until proven otherwise.

Where is the pt from and where did he/she grow up?
The risk of developing MS increases with increasing latitude. Incidence of MS is higher in Canada and northern U.S. than southern U.S. and equator.
In people who have migrated from a high risk area to low risk area before the age of 15 years old, the risk was similar to that of low risk area; whereas in persons who had immigrated after that age, the risk was similar to that of their birthplace.

Is there a family history of MS?
Risk is 25 times higher than normal population if a relative has MS.

Is there any bladder symptoms?
Incontinence and urinary retention are very common in MS. Always ask about urinary tract infection symptoms as it can worsen preexisting MS symptoms.

Perform a general physical and neurologic exam
Common ocular findings include: decreased visual acuity, central scotoma, color desaturation, optic disk atrophy or inflammation, afferent pupillary defect, and internuclear ophthalmoplegia (see chapter on Diplopia).
Check for evidence of spasticity and hyperreflexia, clonus, Babinski's sign, Hoffman sign.
Check for sensory level, loss of positional sense.
Lhermitte's sign is sudden sensation of electric shock down spine and arm when pt flexes neck. It's caused by lesion in high cervical spinal cord.

Obtain MRI of the area of interest with and without contrast
New plaques will enhance with contrast due to inflammation and breakdown of blood-brain barrier.
Old plaques appears as "black holes" on T1-weighted image.
Plaques on corpus callosum on sagittal cut is pathognomic for MS (*Dawson's fingers*).

Obtain evoked potential (EP) testing
Visual EP assesses the integrity of optic nerves. Brainstem auditory EP assesses the auditory pathway from cochlea to inferior colliculus. Somatosensory EP assesses the integrity of spinal cord. These tests are abnormal in 50% to 70% of MS pts even without clinical signs.

Perform lumbar puncture
Check for blood cell count, glucose, protein, and "MS panel," which include myelin basic protein, oligoclonal band, and IgG index and synthesis rate.

Multiple sclerosis
It's estimated approximately 500,000 people have MS in the U.S. The cause is unknown, but has both genetic and environmental factors.
It is a recurrent inflammatory disease of the CNS characterized by attack of T cells on oligodendrocytes in brain and spinal cord. Oligodendrocyte produces myelin in the CNS and the basic pathology is demyelination.

Schwann cells produce myelin in peripheral nerve system and is not affected.
Definition is two or more neurologic symptoms separated by space and time.
There are four clinical courses of MS:
1. Relapse-remitting MS (RRMS)
   - Most common type of MS.
   - Characterized by self-limited attacks of neurologic dysfunction. These attacks develop acutely, evolving over days to weeks.
   - Over the next several weeks to months, most pts experience a recovery of function that is often but not always complete.
   - Between attacks pt is asymptomatic and neurologically stable.
2. Secondary progressive MS
   - Begins as RRMS, but at some point, the attack rate is reduced and the course becomes characterized by a steady deterioration in function unrelated to acute attacks.
3. Primary progressive MS
   - Characterized by a steady decline in function from the beginning without acute attacks.
4. Progressive/relapsing MS
   - Also begins with a progressive course although these pts also experience occasional attacks.

Heat (Uhtoff's sign), infection, fatigue, and tension cause worsening of preexisting symptoms.

Treat acute MS attack or exacerbation
Steroids have been shown to hasten the speed and degree of recovery of neurologic function in acute attacks. However, the long-term benefit remains unclear.
Ensure pt has no evidence of infection (afebrile with normal urinalysis and CXR).
Start high-dose steroid, Solumedrol 1 g IV QD for 3 to 5 days followed by PO prednisone taper over 7 to 14 days.
Supplement potassium with K-Dur 40 meq PO QD.
GI prophylaxis with Zantac, Pepcid, or Prevacid.
Monitor blood sugar with finger sticks and insulin sliding scale.

Start patient on one of the disease-modifying therapies
Avonex, Betaseron, Copaxone, and Rebif are available options.
Avonex, Betaseron, and Rebif are interferons that downregulate TH1 cell function.
Copaxone is a polypeptide that upregulates TH2 cell function.
All four drugs have the same end result—minimize attack of T cells on CNS oligodendrocytes, which translates into fewer MS attacks and better functional capacity.

Engage pt in physical and occupational therapy program
Will hasten recovery from the acute attack. It is important for wheelchair or bedbound MS pt to engage in a physical therapy program to prevent development of contracture and spasticity.

XII
Movement Disorder

Does the pt have *tremor*?
Tremor is the most common presentation in Parkinson's Disease(PD) (~ 70% of pts). Tremor is resting in nature and asymmetric. It most commonly affects the hands but can affect any part of body including legs, trunk, head, and neck. The tremor should subside with intentional use, if it does not, consider other diagnosis such as essential tremor or cerebellar disease.

Does the pt have symptoms of *bradykinesia*?
Like tremor, bradykinesia can affect anywhere but most commonly the hand. Symptoms include micrographia (writing becomes smaller), difficulty using fork and knife, slowness getting up from chair or out of bed, slower walking.

Does pt have symptoms of *rigidity*?
Pt may complain of stiffness in arms and legs, difficulty turning in bed.

Does the pt have *postural instability*?
Difficulty with ambulation with frequent falls. It is usually a late sign of PD. If it occurs early, consider a different diagnosis, such as one of the Parkinson Plus syndromes.

Assess mental status
Perform a mini-mental status exam. Pts with early PD usually have a normal mental status exam. If dementia is a prominent feature at the start of PD symptoms, then consider other diagnosis such as Lewy body dementia.
Note facial expression. PD pts commonly have "mask faces."

Check extraocular movement
↓ vertical gazes raises possibility of progressive supranuclear palsy (PSP).

Evaluate the tremor
Ask pt to sit in a chair with hands resting on the laps and observe for any tremor. Note the amplitude, frequency, and locations of the tremor.
Ask pt to recite the months of year backward. Anxiety increases tremor.
PD pts may have postural tremor that is referred to as a "reemergent" tremor. Ask pt to raise arms to postural position. There will be a brief period when there is no tremor followed by a crescendo increase of tremor until it appears as a typical resting tremor.

Assess muscle tone for rigidity
Check the tones in wrists, elbows, shoulders, neck, and knees on both sides. Compare the two sides. With PD, asymmetry in tones is expected.
If no rigidity is felt, have pt keep opening and closing one hand while you examine the contralateral limb. This maneuver brings out rigidity better.
Cogwheel rigidity can be observed when tremor and rigidity are present in the same arm.

Observe gait
Note the stride. PD pts often take small, shuffling steps.
The arm swing may be decreased on one side. Hand tremor usually becomes more prominent when walking.
Observe how the pt turns. Often they have en bloc turning (i.e., no truncal rotation) and may take many more steps than normal.

Evaluate postural instability
Stand behind the pt and ask him or her to try to stand still. Give the pt a pull on the shoulders backward. Normal pt will not budge or will take one to two steps backward and not fall. PD pts will lose balance and fall easily.

Consider laboratory and imaging studies
PD is a clinical diagnosis. Studies are only needed when there is suspicion regarding secondary cause of PD (e.g., Wilson's disease, strokes).

Parkinson's Disease
PD is not common. One percent of the population older than 50 has PD.
It is uncommon in pts younger than 40 years of age. For these pts, more workup is needed to exclude secondary cause of PD symptoms.
It is caused by the loss of dopaminergic neurons in the substantia nigra and resultant dopamine deficiency in the striatum. The mechanism of cell loss involves formation of *Lewy bodies*, which are cytoplasmic inclusions consisted of abnormally aggregated neurofilament, ubiquitin, and α-*synuclein*.
Function of α-synuclein is unknown. There is a rare familial PD resulting from α-synuclein mutation on chromosome 4. Affected pts get PD symptoms in teenage years.
There are a number of conditions that resemble PD:
- Drugs (mainly anti-emetics and anti-psychotics).
- Toxins such as MPTP (a component in synthetic heroin) and manganese.
- Parkinson plus syndromes (see p. 126).
- Dementias such as Lewy body and Alzheimer's disease.
- Strokes affecting basal ganglia.
- Essential tremor.
- Wilson's disease.

Start medical therapy
Treatment of PD is very individualized and requires expertise. One has to take into account the age, co-morbid conditions, pt's goals and expectation. The two most commonly used starting medications are:
- Dopamine agonists (pramipexole, ropinirole, and pergolide): They are now the usual first-line therapy for PD. They are not as potent as carbidopa/levodopa but dyskinesia is less likely to develop.
- Carbidopa/levodopa: Levodopa is a precursor of dopamine and carbidopa prevents breakdown of levodopa peripherally so more levodopa can enter CNS. It is the most effective medication for PD. However, dyskinesia will develop and can be debilitating. Start in pts who have failed dopamine-agonist or in older pts with limited life span. Other side effects include hypotension and hallucination.

Other medications used include MAO-B inhibitors, bromocriptine, amantadine, anti-cholinergics, and COMT inhibitors.
Most PD pts have very good response to dopamine medications. If symptoms do not improve, one should consider other diagnoses.

Consider surgical options
Deep brain stimulator, pallidotomy, and thalamotomy are the available options. They are reserved for pts who have failed medical therapy or in whom unmanageable dyskinesia developed.

Did the pt respond to levodopa/carbidopa?
Parkinson plus syndromes are difficult to diagnose. Majority of the pts were initially misdiagnosed with Parkinson's disease (PD) and treated with levodopa/carbidopa. Lack of response to the medication should raise suspicion of Parkinson plus syndrome.

Does the pt have hallucination or dementia?
Presence of hallucination and cognitive decline early in the disease suggests Lewy body dementia. The mental status may fluctuate from day to day.

Does the pt have any eye symptoms?
Blepharospasm, difficulty with eye opening and closure, and restricted vertical gazes are features of progressive supranuclear palsy (PSP).

Does the pt have any autonomic symptoms?
Postural dizziness, urinary incontinence, urinary retention, and dry mouth are suggestive of multiple system atrophy (MSA).

 Check orthostatic blood pressure
Measure blood pressure with pt lying, sitting, and standing 2 minutes apart. A decrease of 20 mm Hg systolic or 10 mm Hg diastolic is positive for orthostatic hypotension.
Orthostatic hypotension is suggestive of MSA. Keep in mind pt with PD on levodopa/carbidopa may have drug-induced orthostatic hypotension.

Observe facial features
Pts with PSP often have a characteristic wide-eyed, unblinking stare that looks as if he/she is perpetually surprised.

Assess extraocular muscles
Vertical gaze palsy strongly supports diagnosis of PSP.
Presence of abnormal nystagmus may be seen in PSP and MSA.

Perform Parkinson's disease exam (see PD, p. 124)
All the pts with Parkinson plus syndromes have some features of PD. Tone, tremor, and postural stability should all be tested.

Check for limb apraxia
Apraxia is a motor disorder in which volitional or voluntary movement is impaired without muscle weakness. It is often seen in pts with parietal lobe lesion. Apraxia may be in limb, oral, speech, and gait.

Apraxia is a feature in corticobasal ganglionic degeneration (CBGD). Ask pt to pretend to comb hair or light a match and apraxic pt will be unable to do so. Pt may also have apraxia in walking and sitting. In extreme cases, "alien hand" is seen. Pt does not recognize and cannot control the affected hand. For example, pt may be buttoning a shirt with the good hand, and the "alien hand" may try to hold the good hand or slap pt on the face.

Check for frontal release signs
These are primitive reflexes seen in infants and pts with frontal lobe lesions/atrophy resulting in loss of inhibition. They include palmomental, grasp, snout, root, and suck reflex. (See Dementia, p. 133.)

Check for pyramidal (upper motor neuron) signs
Such as ↑ tone and deep tendon reflexes. Strength may or may not be decreased.

Obtain MRI of brain with contrast
Parkinson plus syndromes usually have unremarkable MRI findings except for atrophy in the selected areas.

Parkinson plus syndromes
"Parkinson plus" is a name given to be a group of neurodegenerative disorders with parkinsonian signs and symptoms, but with different pathology and additional features. There are four major types.
1. **Multiple system atrophy (MSA):** Multiple segments in the nervous system are involved and undergo abnormal degeneration. There are three main subtypes of MSA:
   a. Shy-Drager syndrome: Characterized by disorder/atrophy of *autonomic nervous system*. Pts have orthostatic hypotension, impotence, loss of sweating, dry mouth, miosis, urinary incontinence/retention, and vocal cord palsy.
   b. Striatonigral degeneration: Characterized by disorder/atrophy of *substantia nigra and striatum* (putamen and caudate nucleus). Pts have signs and symptoms very similar to those of PD.
   c. Olivopontocerebellar atrophy: Characterized by disorder/atrophy of the *cerebellum, pons, and olives*. Pts have ataxia, dysarthria, dysphagia, and hyperreflexia.

The previous three diseases were initially described as separate entities but later grouped together under MSA. Pt may have features from one, two, or all three entities. They share the same pathology in which *glial cytoplasmic inclusion* bodies were found in the oligodendroglial cells.

2. **Progressive supranuclear palsy:** Characterized by degeneration of pretectal area, periaqueductal gray, subthalamic nucleus, and superior colliculus. It is one of the *tauopathies* in which abnormally phosphorylated tau proteins are present in the neurons. Tau is a component of a microtubule-associated protein that is responsible for axonal transport of vesicles. Pts present in their 60s and 70s with frequent falls due to postural instability and vertical gaze paresis. They also have features of PD with rigidity and bradykinesia.
3. **Corticobasal ganglionic degeneration:** Another tauopathy involving the frontal and parietal cortex and the extrapyramidal system. Pts present in their 60s with parkinsonian features involving mainly one limb along with apraxia. The limb may resemble "alien hand." The symptom eventually spreads bilaterally with severe disability.
4. **Dementia with Lewy bodies:** Pts present with Alzheimer-like dementia and parkinsonian features. Vivid visual hallucinations are common. Rapid eye movement sleep disorders are common as well.

Again, these Parkinson plus syndromes share common cardinal features of PD including tremor (usually less prominent), rigidity, bradykinesia, and postural instability. It is the additional features of each disease that separate them clinically.

Educate and inform pt of their likely diagnosis
In general, Parkinson plus syndromes do not respond well to PD medications. No cure is available. Pts eventually progress to severe disability and die within 8 to 10 yrs. Pts see, on average, three to five neurologists before being given the correct diagnosis. The physician should help pts understand and cope with their illness. Treatment is symptomatic and supportive.

S

Where is the tremor?
Most often the tremor is present in the arms. They are symmetric, but in 15% of cases, it involves only the dominant hand.
Tremor can also affect the legs, head, jaws, lips, tongue, and larynx, causing quavering voice.

How are the activities of daily living affected?
Try to understand how the tremor is causing disability for the pt. This will help to decide whether or not to treat with medications.

When does the tremor occur?
Tremors can be divided into two major categories, action and resting. Most of the tremors, including essential tremor, are action tremor. They occur when muscle is in motion or maintaining posture. Pts often complain tremor is worse with writing, eating, and holding cup.
If the tremor occurs at rest and goes away with action, then it is more likely to be Parkinson's disease (PD).
If tremor is present only when standing and is predominantly in the legs, then pt is likely to have *orthostatic tremor*.

What makes the tremor better and what makes it worse?
With essential tremor, the tremor is typically worse with anxiety, fright, exercise, fatigue, and α-adrenergic medications.
It is usually better with EtOH and relaxation.

Ask about alcohol and sedative use
Withdrawal from EtOH and sedatives such as benzodiazepines and barbiturates cause tremor that is very similar to essential tremor.

Is pt taking medications that can cause tremor?
Common medications that cause tremor include valproic acid, tricyclics, thyroxine, lithium, prednisone, neuroleptics, antiemetics, amiodarone, atorvastatin, bronchodilators, caffeine, cyclosporine, SSRI, metronidazole, methylxanthines, and β-adrenergic agonists.

Is there a family history of tremor?
Essential tremor is often genetic (>60%) and is inherited in autosomal dominant manner. When family history is positive, it is called *familial tremor*. If family history is negative, then it is called *essential tremor*. If the tremor starts in late adult life, then it is called *senile tremor*.
By comparison, PD pts usually have a negative family history.

Rule out Parkinson's disease
Essential tremor is a diagnosis by exclusion. Other causes of tremor should be excluded (see subsequent section) (see PD, p. 124).
Pts with essential tremor DO NOT have rigidity, bradykinesia, and postural instability.
Essential tremor primarily involves hands, head, and voice whereas PD tremor occurs in hands, legs, and perioral area.
Tremor in face, tongue, or jaw is likely due to PD, while a head tremor is more typical of essential tremor.
Essential tremor is of kinetic and postural type. Resting tremor is one of the cardinal features of PD.

Rule out cerebellar cause of tremor
Cerebellar and midbrain lesions cause tremors as well and physician must be able to recognize the difference.

Ask pt to do finger-nose test and observe the tremor. *Cerebellar intention tremor* is absent at rest and at early part of voluntary movement. As pt's finger moves closer to the target and requires fine adjustments, the tremor can be seen. The tremor is oscillatory and occurs in more than one plane, unlike essential tremor. The side of the tremor is ipsilateral to the side of cerebellar lesion.

Lesions in the red nucleus of midbrain cause *rubral tremor*. Rubral tremor is a violent, high-amplitude, "wing-beating" movement that is present with *every* movement of the arm, ranging from lifting the arm slightly to maintaining it in fixed posture.

Lesion in the midline cerebellum can cause *titubation*, which is a rhythmic tremor of the head and upper trunk mostly in the anteroposterior plane.

Sometimes these tremors due to cerebellar disease can be difficult to diagnose.

Therefore, it is important to look for other signs of cerebellar and brainstem dysfunction. Carefully assess extraocular muscles, nystagmus, hypotonia, and gait ataxia.

Perform maneuvers to bring out essential tremor

Have pt raise and maintain both arms outstretched in front. This should markedly enhance the tremor if it is essential in nature.

Have pt write a sentence and draw Archimedes spirals. These are objective tests the physician can use to follow the pt. Keep a record in the chart.

Essential Tremor

It is the most common movement disorder affecting approximately 5 million Americans and 10% of individuals older than age 65.

It may start as early as childhood years and persist throughout life. The incidence goes up as age increases. Men and women are affected equally.

Pathophysiology is not known and there is no obvious pathologic abnormality associated.

Differential diagnosis includes PD, enhanced physiologic tremor, drug-induced tremor, metabolic disease (see subsequent section), cerebellar tremors, orthostatic tremor, and neuropathic tremor, dystonic tremor, and psychogenic tremor.

Tremor can be caused by metabolic diseases such as hyperthyroidism, hyperparathyroidism, hypocalcemia, hyponatremia, and Wilson's disease.

Decide whether pt needs treatment

Not all pts with essential tremor need to be treated. Discuss with pt. The disability has to be great enough for pt to be willing to take medication every day.

Start propranolol or primidone

Propranolol 10 mg PO BID and titrate up to maximum 320 mg/day.

Alternatively, primidone 25 mg PO QHS and titrate up to maximum of 250 mg/day. They are effective in treating essential tremor 75% of the time.

Consider surgical options

Only in severe cases. Thalamotomy and thalamic deep brain stimulation are available options.

XIII
Neurodegenerative Disease

What is the time course?
Dementia is a chronic condition. If demented symptoms develop acutely, it is delirium.

Does pt have memory loss?
Memory loss is the earliest manifestation of Alzheimer's disease (AD).
Pts have difficulties finding things, remembering recent conversations or events, asking same questions repeatedly, and missing appointments.

Does the pt have decreased language facility?
Language expressions become less precise. Circumlocution and perseveration are common.
Later in the disease, conversation may become slowed and less spontaneous.

Does the pt have visual spatial dysfunction?
They have problem finding a parked car in the parking lot. Many will lose a sense of direction and get lost especially when traveling an unfamiliar route.

Does the pt have symptoms of apraxia?
Pt will have lost the ability to carry out everyday activities, such as dressing, tying shoes, unlocking a door with a key, and starting a car.

Does the pt have symptoms of frontal lobe dysfunction?
With *orbitofrontal* involvement, pt may be disinhibited with socially inappropriate behaviors without showing any concern, overactive, restless, and have a fatuous affect.
With *dorsolateral* prefrontal involvement, pt may be apathetic and inert, lacking in drive and initiative and minimally responsive to external stimuli.
They may become increasingly apathetic and lose interest in reading, watching TV, and social gathering.
Less attention is paid to grooming and tidiness. They may become sloppily dressed. The house may become untidy and disorganized.
Personality and behavior change early in the disease and is more consistent with frontotemporal dementia (FTD) and Pick's disease.

Are there symptoms of parkinsonism?
Parkinsonism may develop at later stages in patients with AD.
If Parkinson symptoms develop early with cognitive impairment, consider diffuse Lewy body disease as the diagnosis.

Look for symptoms of depression
Although demented pts are often depressed, depression itself can cause "pseudodementia," which resolves when depression is treated.

Perform a general physical exam
Pay attention to signs of endocrine disease such as thyroid, Cushing's.
Sign of malnutrition, chronic alcoholism.
Signs of malignancy, cachexia.

Perform a complete mental status evaluation
Insight: does pt have insight to his/her illness? Ask what can I do for you? Why are you here? When did your illness begin?
Orientation: Person, place, and time.
Memory: For recent memory, perform 5-minute recall on three words such as "chair, pipe, and honesty." Make sure the pt is able to *register* by repeating it immediately.
Language: For verbal language, the most important parts to test are fluency, comprehension, and repetition. Also test reading and writing.
Concentration: Do serial 7, "world/dlrow," or recite months of year backward.

Visual spatial: Have pt draw a clock, bicycle, or house. Check for angulation, organization, and symmetry.
Mini-Mental Status Examination: Is a quick and easy way to screen for dementia. A score of 24 or less is suggestive of dementia.

Look for frontal release signs
These are primitive reflexes that are present in infants but are inhibited as the frontal lobe matured. They are present in frontal lobe diseases.
Grasp reflex: Gently slide your hand in pt's palm and pt will try to grasp your hand.
Snout: Gently tap the lips; causes pouting of the lips.
Root: Gently stroke the lateral upper lip causes the mouth to move toward the same side.
Palmomental: Stroking the palm of the hand will cause the ipsilateral mentalis muscle of the lower lip to contract.

Perform remainder of neurologic exam
Cranial nerves, motor, sensory, cerebellar, and gait.

Send for laboratory studies
Chemistry, CBC, thyroid-stimulating hormone (TSH), rapid plasma reagin, vitamin B_{12}, urinalysis, HIV to look for treatable causes of dementia.

Order EEG
Demented pts show generalized slowing of brain activity on EEG.
Huntington's disease gives a very low voltage background.
Continuous partial subclinical status epilepticus is also ruled out by EEG.

Obtain MRI of the brain
Mainly to exclude structural and potentially reversible cases such as subdural hematoma, hydrocephalus, strokes, and tumor.
Look for pattern of atrophy. AD causes the most atrophy in the hippocampus, hippocampal formation, amygdala, thalamus, and anterior temporal lobe.
Frontotemporal dementia and Pick's disease has strikingly more atrophy in the frontal and temporal lobes.

Obtain neuropsychological testing
It is an extensive cognitive test done by behavior neurologist or psychiatrists. It evaluates in detail various brain functions, including visual-spatial, language, memory, planning, attention.
The data are then analyzed and a neuroanatomic localization is formulated (e.g., frontal vs. parietal, cortical vs. subcortical, right vs. left).
It is helpful in establishing the exact diagnosis of dementia (e.g., AD, frontotemporal dementia, progressive supranuclear palsy).

Dementia
The following are the most common dementias listed in order of frequency.

Alzheimer's disease
Affects > 10% of population > 65 yrs of age and 25% of population > 80.
Onset is usually 50 to 65 yrs of age. Women are affected two to three times more often than men.
Approximately 15% of AD cases are familial. Chromosome 21 abnormalities are associated with AD. AD develops in almost all pts with Down's syndrome (trisomy 21) if they live to be older than 30 years. Amyloid precursor protein gene (on chromosome 21) mutation causes autosomal dominant AD.
Chromosomes 14 and 1 carries the presenillin 1 and 2 protein, respectively. Mutation of these genes causes autosomal dominant AD.

Homozygosity of the E4 allele of apolipoprotein E (on chromosome 19) confers an increased risk for AD.

Neurofibrillary tangles, senile plaques, and *granulovacuolar degenerations* are the main pathologic feature of AD. Neuronal death occurs as these accumulate in cells and interfere with normal cell function.

Neuronal cell death at basal nucleus of Meynert causes reduction in cerebral acetylcholine. This is the basis for using central choline esterase inhibitors in treatment of AD.

Clinical deterioration of cognitive functions occurs progressively to the point of being bedridden without meaningful interactive ability. Course is 3 to 12 years. Death is usually caused by infections from pneumonia, urosepsis, or decubitus ulcer.

Vascular dementia

Focal strokes involving various regions of the brain (particularly nondominant parietal lobe, temporal lobe) can cause dementia-like symptoms. Diagnosis is not difficult because symptoms occur acutely.

Diagnosis is more difficult in multi-infarct dementia. Pts usually have history of minor strokes (hemiparesis, ataxia, diplopia) with recovery of symptoms. The cognition declines gradually over time.

When the strokes are predominantly *subcortical* (lacunar infarcts in corona radiate, internal capsule, thalamus), predominant symptoms are psychomotor retardation, inertia, and decreased attention and concentration.

When strokes are predominantly *cortical*, symptoms are aphasia, apraxia, amnesia, and visual-spatial disturbances.

Lewy body dementia

The clinical picture lies somewhere between AD and Parkinson's disease.

Pts present initially with parkinsonism, which is nonresponsive to traditional PD meds. Visual hallucination occurs early too. Later pt develops ↓ cognition that may fluctuate with "good days" and "bad days."

Like PD, Lewy bodies are seen microscopically and are consisted of mainly α-synuclein. Like AD, neurofibrillary tangles, senile plaques, and granulovacuolar degenerations are seen.

There is cell loss in substantia nigra like PD and basal nucleus of Meynert neurons similar to AD.

Frontotemporal dementia and Pick's disease

Unlike AD, the earliest manifestation is loss of frontal inhibition of socially unacceptable behavior. Language is affected early as well. Memory impairment is not as prominent.

At autopsy, the most striking feature is "knife-edge" cortical atrophy involving the frontal and temporal region with sparing of the posterior two thirds of superior temporal gyrus and the rest of brain.

FTD and Pick's disease are differentiated only at autopsy. Pick bodies (intraneuronal cytoplasmic filamentous inclusions that contain predominantly tau protein) are present in Pick's disease but not in FTD.

Other primary neurodegenerative diseases causing dementia

Include PD, Parkinson plus syndromes, Huntington's disease, progressive aphasia.

Secondary causes of dementia

Infections: HIV, subacute sclerosing panencephalitis, rubella, Creutzfeldt-Jakob virus, syphilis, Lyme, TB, cryptococcus, Whipple's disease.

Metabolic: hypothyroidism, vitamin deficiencies, Cushing's, hyperparathyroidism and hypoparathyroidism, chronic renal failure, cirrhosis, Wilson's disease, mitochondrial diseases, certain inborn errors of metabolism that occur in early or middle adult life (metachromatic leukodystrophy, ceroid-lipofuscinosis, adrenoleukodystrophy, adult polyglucosan body disease).
Drugs and toxins: EtOH, barbiturate, arsenic, mercury, and toluene.
Depression (pseudodementia).
Normal pressure hydrocephalus.

Treat the reversible causes of dementia

Always screen for the reversible causes first when evaluating demented pts.

Start treatment
Cholinesterase inhibitors slow the progression of AD and delay admission to chronic nursing facility. Most physicians prescribe them for the other types of dementia as well. The available meds include: donepezil, tacrine, rivastigmine, memantine, and galantamine.
Start vitamin E 1000 I.U. PO BID.
Selegiline and ginkgo biloba may be considered but real evidence is lacking.

Treat other psychiatric aspects of demented pts
Depression, agitation, and psychosis are very common.
Atypical antipsychotics should be used for agitation and psychosis.
Selected tricyclics, MAO-B inhibitors, and SSRIs can be used for depression.

Educate family and caregiver
There are many programs in the community that provide education of caring for demented pts. They can improve caregiver satisfaction and delay time to nursing home placement.

Behavior modification
Scheduled toileting and prompt voiding can reduce urinary incontinence.
Graded assistance, practice, and positive enforcement should be used to increase functional independence.
Intensive multimodality group training may improve activities of daily living.
Low lighting levels, music, and simulated nature sounds may improve eating behavior.
Walking or other forms of light exercise may decrease behavior problems.
Hang calendars at different places to improve orientation.

XIV
Sleep Disorders

S **Does the pt have excessive daytime sleepiness (EDS)?**
EDS is the primary symptom of narcolepsy. Pt feels sleepy most times of the day. The sleepiness causes pt to fall asleep without warning (i.e., sleep attacks) during passive activities (e.g., watching TV). In severe cases, the sleep attacks can occur during activities such as walking and driving.
A widely used questionnaire to assess EDS is the Epworth Sleepiness scale.
- Using a scale of 0 to 3, with 0 being never and 3 being very likely, ask the patient how often he/she will fall asleep under the following situations?
  1. Sitting and reading.
  2. Watching TV.
  3. Sitting and being inactive in a public place.
  4. Riding as passenger in a car for 1 hour without break.
  5. Lying down to rest in the afternoon when circumstances permit.
  6. Sitting and talking to someone.
  7. Sitting quietly after a lunch without alcohol.
  8. In a car, while stopped for a few minutes in traffic.
- Score > 10 warrants an investigation. Score > 16 indicates severe EDS.

Does pt have cataplexy?
Cataplexy is sudden loss of muscle tone brought about by emotions such as laughter fear, anger, and excitement. Approximately 70% of narcoleptic pts have cataplexy.
If mild, pt may complain of jaw sagging, head dropping, and tongue paralyzing, or dropping things from hand.
In severe cases, pt may complain of knee buckling, falling, and becoming completely paralyzed. Pt usually will be able to avoid injury by finding support before fall.
Symptoms usually lasts seconds to minutes during which consciousness is preserved but pt might not be able to speak or open eyes due to muscle weakness. Cataplexy may last longer if pt goes to sleep.

Does pt sometimes have hallucinations falling asleep or waking up?
The hallucination is mostly *hypnagogic* (going from wake to sleep state) but can be *hypnopompic* (going from sleep to wake state). Approximately 30% of narcoleptic pts have it.
The hallucinations are mostly visual but can be auditory, tactile, or gustatory in nature. Pt may report seeing colored circles, animals, or persons. They may hear bell ringing and voices. They may also feel rubbing, touching, or sense of levitation like an out-of-body experience.
What distinguishes hypnagogic hallucination from dreams is timing. Hypnagogic hallucination occurs immediately when pt goes into sleep state. Dreaming occurs during rapid eye movement (REM) sleep, which occurs later in sleep.

Does the pt sometimes have sleep paralysis?
Sleep paralysis can be either hypnagogic or hypnopompic. Approximately 40% of narcoleptic pts have sleep paralysis.
Pt is awake and conscious during the episode but is unable to perform even the smallest movements such as opening their eyes or lifting a finger.

Perform a general and neurologic exam
Mainly to rule out other causes for pt's problem. Pts with narcolepsy should have a normal exam.

Consider sleep studies
Narcolepsy is a clinical diagnosis. If pt has EDS and cataplexy, no other workup is needed. If diagnosis is questionable, then obtain sleep studies.

Overnight polysomnography (see next chapter) and next-day multiple sleep latency test are the gold standard.

Narcolepsy

Prevalence is approximately 60 per 100,000 people. Onset is at 15 to 30 y/o. Men and women are affected equally.

To understand narcolepsy, one has to learn the normal stages of sleep.
- Awake: characterized by EEG α rhythm of 8.5 to 12 Hz with eyes closed.
- Stage 1 (drowsiness): EEG changes to lower voltage and frequencies with loss of α waves. Slow rolling eye movements are present.
- Stage 2 sleep: sleep spindles (biparietal 12 to 14 Hz burst activities) and K complexes (sharp slow-waves) can be seen.
- Stages 3 and 4 sleep: characterized by increasing portion of slow δ (1 to 2 Hz) waves. These are the deep stages of sleep.
- Stage 5 (REM) sleep: EEG becomes desynchronized with low-voltage and high-frequency discharge pattern. There is loss of muscle tone in the body except extraocular muscles, which gives rise to bursts of REMs.

In normal adults, sleep involves passing successively through stages 1, 2, 3, and 4 of sleep (non-REM stages). This process takes approximately 90 to 120 minutes after which REM sleep starts and lasts anywhere from 10 to 60 minutes.

The non-REM–REM cycle then starts over again and repeats throughout sleep. Toward the latter part of sleep, the duration of REM sleep increases and the duration of stages 3 to 4 sleep decreases. As people age, the time spent in stages 3 to 4 decreases.

In narcolepsy patients, sleep latency (time it takes to enter stage 1 sleep) and REM sleep latency (time from sleep onset to REM) are reduced to an abnormally short time. REM sleep can occur immediately at sleep onset.

Cataplexy, hypnagogic hallucination, and sleep paralysis are all phenomenon of REM sleep.

Differential diagnosis to consider includes other sleep disorders, syncope, and seizures.

Advise good sleep hygiene

Do not take naps. Avoid caffeine, EtOH, nicotine, and strenuous exercise before sleep. Use bed only for sleep and sex. Sleep only when sleepy. Get up and go to bed at the same time everyday. Take a hot bath 90 minutes before sleep. Make the bed and bedroom as comfortable as possible.

Treat EDS

Stimulants such as amphetamine derivatives (dextroamphetamine and methamphetamine) and methylphenidate enhance the release and inhibit the reuptake of catecholamines. They have high addictive potential.

Modafinil is a new drug with unknown mechanism but has lower addictive potential.

Monoamine oxidase (MAO) inhibitors and L-dopa have been shown to be effective.

β-hydroxybutyrate (a.k.a., date-rape drug) given at night to promote full sleep is another strategy to treat EDS.

Treat cataplexy, hypnagogic hallucination, and sleep paralysis

Tricyclics (clomipramine, imipramine, desipramine, protriptyline) are the most effective agents because they are potent REM sleep inhibitors.

SSRIs, MAO inhibitor are alternatives if pt cannot tolerate tricyclics.

Obstructive Sleep Apnea

S **Does the pt have excessive daytime sleepiness?**
EDS is the major symptom of obstructive sleep apnea (OSA). Refer to Narcolepsy, p. 138.

Does the pt have night symptoms of OSA?
Almost all will have long history of loud snoring.
Pt may complain of difficulty falling asleep and frequent awakening during night.
Sometimes choking and sitting up gasping for air may be reported.
Spouse will often witness apnea. This strongly support the diagnosis.

Does the pt have risk factors for OSA?
Male gender, increasing age > 40, and obesity.

Does the pt have chronic medical conditions associated with OSA?
Hypertension, cardiac arrhythmia, congestive heart failure (CHF), myocardial infarction, stroke, and pulmonary hypertension. These conditions often improve after successful treatment of OSA.

O **Perform a general and neurologic exam**
Measure height and weight to obtain body mass index. Seventy percent of patients with OSA are obese.
Neck circumference > 17 inches for men and 16 inches for women is associated with OSA.
Examine the oropharynx and look for low-hanging soft palate, large uvula, and large tonsils (especially in kids).
Look for signs of cardiovascular and pulmonary disease.

Obtain sleep studies
Overnight polysomnography (PSG) is diagnostic. PSG consists of EEG, EMG, airflow thermistor, oximetry, ECG, and plethysmography. It records the stages of sleep, muscle movements, air flow, blood oxygen level, and respiratory effort.
Apnea-hypopnea index (AHI) is the number of hypopneic and apneic episodes in 1 hour. AHI > 5 is considered abnormal. Hypoxemia is detected during those episodes.
Once sleep apneas are documented, pt is awakened, connected to continuous positive airway pressure (CPAP) machine, and allowed to sleep. CPAP levels are then titrated up until pt stops experiencing apnea.

A **Obstructive Sleep Apneas**
Sleep apneas include obstructive, central, and mixed. Of these, obstructive sleep apnea is the most common. The prevalence is 4% in men and 2% in women.
Healthy people occasionally experience sleep apneas, especially during REM sleep. To be considered abnormal, there has to be at least five episodes/hr and 10 seconds/episode.
OSA is caused by collapse of the pharyngeal muscles blocking the airway. This is more likely to happen in REM sleep when muscle tone is decreased. Obstruction of airway causes hypoxemia, which wakes up the pt momentarily (pt may not remember). This happens throughout the night causing fragmentation of sleep and daytime EDS. Frequent hypoxemic episodes may be the cause for the cardiovascular complications.
Obese people have more fat in the pharynx and soft palate, and therefore are more prone to OSA.
Central apnea is caused by abnormalities in the brainstem respiratory center. It can be caused by structural lesions, toxic/metabolic, and hypoxia. Cheyne-Stokes is one type of central apnea and may be seen in CHF pts with hypoperfusion to the brainstem.

Differential diagnosis to consider when evaluating pts with EDS:
- Sleep deprivation: the most common cause and is often occupational (e.g., interns and residents).
- Insomnia: the most common sleep disorder, affecting one third of US population at one time or another. Causes may be medical (CHF, peptic ulcer disease, drugs), psychological (depression, mania), or environmental (shift work, jet lag, stress).
- Narcolepsy: see p. 138.
- Upper airway resistance syndrome: similar to OSA, but the airways are not obstructed. Pt has loud snoring and frequent awakenings.
- Restless leg syndrome: a sensorimotor disorder characterized by uncomfortable sensation in the legs, worse when sitting or lying, and relieved with movement (both voluntary and involuntary). Symptoms have circadian variability and are mostly seen when going to bed. Approximately 50% have positive family history with autosomal dominant pattern. Cause is idiopathic but can be associated with iron deficiency, pregnancy, neuropathies, multiple sclerosis, peripheral vascular disease, and caffeine.
- Periodic limb movement disorder (PLMD): has high association with restless leg syndrome (RLS). Characterized by repetitive (every 20 to 40 seconds) leg muscle jerks during non-REM sleep. Treatment with dopaminergic agents (pramipexole, ropinirole, carbidopa/levodopa, pergolide, bromocriptine), benzodiazepines, gabapentin, and opiates are helpful with PLMD and RLS.

P

Lifestyle modification

Weight loss is the most important. Weight reduction in obese patient will improve OSA and decrease other obesity-related health problems.

Avoid EtOH and other sedative-hypnotics.

Raising the head of the bed and avoiding the supine position during sleep may decrease the incidence of apnea. Elevation of the head tends to bring the tongue forward, while sleeping on the side moves the tongue laterally.

Initiate ventilatory support

Nasal CPAP keeps the airway from collapsing. Pt often report dramatic difference in quality of sleep.

For pt unable to tolerate CPAP, bilevel positive airway pressure (BiPAP) may be used. BiPAP delivers higher pressure during inspiration and lower pressure during expiration.

Nasal pillow or facial mask can be tried if pt cannot tolerate nasal mask.

Make effort to work with pt to find the best ventilatory support. Compliance is the major hindrance to successful OSA treatment.

Consider referral to ENT or oral surgery

Chronic rhinitis, nasal polyps, and septal deviation reduce nasal airflow and worsen OSA.

Uvulopalatopharyngoplasty has an approximate 50% response rate in OSA.

In children, tonsillectomy and adenoidectomy may be helpful.

Pts with maxillomandibular anatomy that predisposes them to airway obstruction may be considered for special denture or jaw surgery.

XV
Pediatric Neurology

Floppy Baby Syndrome

S **Obtain detailed prenatal, perinatal and family history**
Any medication, illicit drug, infection during pregnancy?
Any family member with neuromuscular or other neurologic disease?

Does the baby have any other symptoms besides being floppy?
Mental retardation and seizures suggest cerebral involvement.
Difficulty breathing may suggest muscular or neuromuscular problem.

Ask about developmental history
Babies who have previous normal development and suddenly develop hypotonia need more urgent evaluation. Possible causes include sepsis, meningitis, hypothyroidism, botulism, and poisoning.

O **Observe and maneuver the infant**
Hypotonic infants have very little spontaneous movements. Legs are fully abducted laying on the bed. Arms are extended and laying on the bed.
Dysmorphic feature may be sign of brain malformation.
Hip dislocation and arthrogryposis (joint contracture) are results of intrauterine immobilization.
Do traction response. Grab the hands and pull the infant to a sitting position. The weakness of neck flexors will cause head to drop back.
Do vertical suspension. Hold the baby up under axilla without grasping the thorax. Because of weak shoulder muscles, the infant may slip through examiner's hands. The head will fall forward and legs dangle.
Do horizontal suspension. Lift the baby under abdomen. Normal baby should maintain an erect posture while hypotonic baby hangs like rag doll.

Determine where the weakness is coming from

Is the weakness central or peripheral?

- CNS: mental retardation, decreased consciousness, seizures, spasticity, brisk reflexes, clonus, dystonia, choreoathetosis.
- Peripheral nerves, neuromuscular junction, muscle: atrophy, fasciculation, decreased reflexes.

Send for laboratory studies
Chemistry, Ca, Mg, CBC, creatine kinase, thyroid-stimulating hormone, blood culture, ammonia, lactate, pyruvate, urine organic acids.

Consider lumbar puncture
Is done as a screening test to rule out meningitis and clues to other CNS or metabolic disease.

Consider EMG and nerve conduction study (NCS)
If the exam is consistent with peripheral process, EMG will differentiate between myopathies vs. neuropathies. Myopathies will give brief, small amplitude, abundant polyphasic potentials while neuropathies will show fibrillations, fasciculations, sharp waves, and large, prolonged, and polyphasic motor unit potentials.
Neuropathies can be further evaluated by NCS to distinguish between demyelinating vs. axonal disease. Demyelination shows a slow conduction velocity, while axonal injury causes a decrease in amplitude.
Repetitive stimulation will rule out neuromuscular junction disease.

Consider muscle biopsy
If EMG demonstrates myopathy.

Consider CT, MRI of brain, or scalp ultrasound

If the exam localizes the CNS. It will rule out hypoxic-ischemia, hemorrhage, and malformations. MRI may show abnormalities (e.g., demyelination) resulting from metabolic disorders. Ultrasound is more sensitive in detecting brain abnormality in newborns and is preferred because no sedation is required.

Floppy infant

Very common problem the neurologists are asked to evaluate. The first step in evaluating a hypotonic infant is to determine the source of the weakness through exams and studies. The following is the differential diagnosis based on location affected:

- Brain: hypoxic-ischemic encephalopathy, malformations such as agenesis of corpus callosum and lissencephaly, kernicterus, chromosome disorders (Prader-Willi, trisomy), peroxisomal disorders (Zellweger, adrenoleukodystrophy), inborn error of metabolism (GM1 gangliosidosis, acid maltase deficiency).
- Spinal cord: transection of the cord caused by breech delivery, maldevelopment such as occult spinal dysraphic defects, spinal muscular atrophies.
- Anterior horn cell: Werdnig-Hoffman disease (infantile spinal muscular atrophy).
- Neuropathies: metachromatic leukodystrophy, Krabbe's, hypertrophic neuropathies, familial dysautonomia, infantile neuroaxonal dystrophy, congenital hypomyelinating neuropathy.
- Neuromuscular disorder: botulism, neonatal myasthenia gravis (caused by placental transfer of maternal autoantibody), congenital myasthenia gravis (caused by infant's autoantibodies to various neuromuscular junction proteins).
- Myopathies: centronuclear myopathy, nemaline rod, central core disease, congenital muscular dystrophy, metabolic myopathies (acid maltase, cytochrome-c oxidase, phosphofructokinase, phosphorylase deficiency).

Note that many chromosomal and metabolic disorders will cause hypotonia. Most will have other organ systems affected though. The ones that may manifest only as hypotonia include Pompe's, cytochrome-c oxidase deficiency, phosphofructokinase deficiency, and McArdle disease. Prader-Willi syndrome is characterized by hypotonia, hypogonadism, mental retardation, short stature, and obesity.

Supportive treatment

Many of the metabolic causes can be treated with diet modification and supplements. Most of the causes of infant hypotonia are without cure. Treatment is supportive.

Multidisciplinary approach with physical therapist and orthopedist is helpful.

Special attention should be paid to the hips, feet, and spine. They are likely to develop contractures, fractures, and malformations with time.

S **Does the pt have any symptoms of mitochondrial disorder?**
Mitochondria are present in all cells and provide the basic energy unit, adenosine triphosphate (ATP). Virtually all organs are potential targets.
- Heart: palpitation, heart failure.
- Endocrine: diabetes, polyuria, polydipsia, short stature.
- GI: constipation, malabsorption, weight loss.
- Nervous system:
  - Visual disturbances: double vision, blurry, blindness.
  - Seizures, jerking, involuntary movements.
  - Weakness, exercise intolerance, fatigue.
  - Hearing loss, numbness, headache.
  - Cognitive decline.
  - Unsteadiness.

Obtain detailed family history
Mitochondria DNA is inherited maternally and does not recombine; mutations thus accumulate sequentially through maternal lineages.
Some of the mitochondrial oxidative phosphorylation proteins are transcribed from nuclear DNA, therefore they may exhibit Mendelian pattern (i.e., autosomal dominant or recessive).
Sometimes the maternal relatives may be asymptomatic or have very mild clinical symptoms. Ask about early onset diabetes, hypertension, seizures, developmental delay, weakness, and exercise intolerance.

 Perform comprehensive general physical
Cardiac: palpate for murmurs and arrhythmias, signs of heart failure.
GI: check hepatosplenomegaly, hypoactive bowel sound.
Skin: lipomas with characteristic horse-collar distribution on the thorax.
Hematology: evidence of anemia, pale skin, conjunctivae.
Pulmonary: abnormal rate and pattern of breathing, hypoventilation and hyperventilation.

Perform comprehensive neurologic exam
Mitochondrial disorder can potentially affect the entire neurologic axis from brain to peripheral nerves and muscles.
Ptosis and ophthalmoplegia are seen in progressive external ophthalmoplegia (PEO) and Kearns-Sayre syndrome.
Myoclonus in MELAS.
Decreased visual acuity and optic disk atrophy in Leber's.
Sensorineural hearing loss.
Dementia.
Ataxia.
Peripheral neuropathy.
Dystonia.
Evidence of stroke (hemiparesis, hemisensory loss) suggests MELAS.

Order the following laboratory studies
Comprehensive chemistry panel, CBC with differential, thyroid-stimulating hormone, parathyroid hormone, HgbA1c, lactate, pyruvate, amylase, lipase, ABG, urinalysis, and urine amino acids.
ECG, CXR, brainstem auditory-evoked response or audiogram hearing test, pulmonary function tests.
Perform lumbar puncture and send cerebrospinal fluid for routine studies. Protein, lactate, and pyruvate are elevated as the result of respiratory chain abnormality.

If available, send for biochemical studies on oxidative phosphorylation and DNA tests.

Perform EMG/nerve conduction study (NCS) and muscle biopsy
EMG may show myopathic potentials. NCS may show axonal and demyelinating peripheral neuropathy.
Skeletal muscle biopsy shows *ragged red fibers*, which is the pattern seen in muscle when mitochondria are abnormal. It is "ragged" because the abnormal mitochondria are abundant in number and large inside type 1 (red) muscle fibers. Note that ragged red fibers take years to develop and therefore might be visible in infants and young children.

Consider MRI of brain
Especially if there is any CNS manifestation (stroke, seizure, dementia).
MRI may show basal ganglia calcification, evidences of strokes, and increased signals in thalamus, brainstem, and spinal cord.

There are varieties of mitochondrial disorders
Progressive external ophthalmoplegia: Usually autosomal dominant, but other inheritance patterns are possible. Onset can be in childhood, adolescence, or less commonly, early adulthood. It primarily affects the extraocular muscles, causing ptosis and ophthalmoplegia. There is weakness in both eye opening and closure. Ophthalmoplegia is symmetric and eyes are fixed and conjugated in central position so there is no double vision. Limb myopathy can occur many years afterward.
Kearns-Sayre syndrome: Same as PEO, but begins before 20 year of age and with additional retinitis pigmentosa, ataxia, heart block, and ↑ CSF protein.
Leigh disease: Inheritance can be any pattern but maternal is more common. Onset is usually before the first year but can occur as late as early adulthood. Manifestation varies widely but involves generalized muscle (both cranial and limb) weakness, seizures, myoclonic jerks, developmental delay, respiratory disturbances. MRI shows abnormalities in thalamus, brainstem, and spinal cord.
Neuropathy, Ataxia, and Retinitis Pigmentosa (NARP): Maternally inherited. It's similar to Leigh disease but occurs in early adulthood.
Myopathy, Encephalopathy, Lactic Acidosis, and Strokes (MELAS): Onset is in mid childhood or adolescent. There is normal early development followed by recurrent seizures and strokes which lead to encephalopathy. Many pts have migraine headache. Muscle biopsy shows ragged red fiber.
Myoclonic Epilepsy with Ragged Red Fiber (MERRF): Disease begins in late childhood or early adulthood and presents with myoclonus which can be elicited by movement or startle. Seizures, cerebellar ataxia, and myopathy are other features.

Supplement with elements of electron transport chain
Coenzyme Q10, menadione, phylloquinone, ascorbic acid, idebenone, riboflavin, nicotinamide, dichloroacetate, sodium succinate, creatine, L-carnitine, B complex vitamin, antioxidant are good supplements that pts should take.
Treatment will help reduce symptoms and delay or prevent progression of disease.
Genetic counseling if pt is considering having children.

S **Are there any neurologic symptoms?**
Hearing loss, tinnitus, balance impairment indicate vestibular nerve involvement from acoustic schwannoma in NF2.
Facial weakness may be due to CN7 compression from cerebellopontine angle tumor, most common of which is acoustic schwannoma in NF2.
Seizures suggest intracranial involvement with tumors or angiomas, which is common in Sturge-Weber syndrome (SW) and Tay-Sachs disease (TS).

Are there any vision problems?
Blurry vision, blindness, constricted visual field can be due to optic nerve sheath meningiomas or retina and choroid hamartoma in NF. Early onset cataract is seen in NF2 in pediatric population.

Obtain detailed family history
Many of these syndromes are hereditary. Ask about known diagnosis or neurologic signs and symptoms in the family.

Examine the skin
Facial angiofibromas (adenoma sebaceum) are pink nodules or plaques on the nose, cheeks, chin, forehead, and scalp. They are pathognomonic of TS.
Shagreen patches are pinkish maculopapular skin areas 1 to 10 cm in diameter that have a feel of "orange peel" or "elephant hide." They are located on the trunk, especially lumbosacral area and are pathognomonic of TS.
Axillary and inguinal freckles suggest NF1.
Café au lait spots are hyperpigmented macules > 5 mm in diameter. If the child has more than six spots, then the diagnosis of NF1 can be made.
Various skin nodules and outgrowth are seen in NF1. They may be non-neural tumors (molluscum fibrosum) or subcutaneous neural tumors attached to peripheral nerves.
Port-wine stain is light pink to deep red and purple papular lesion located on the face, specifically trigeminal V1 distribution (upper eyelid, forehead, scalp). It suggests SW.

Perform neurologic exam
Lisch nodules are iris hamartomas best seen using slit-lamp and are pathognomonic of NF1.
Check visual acuity and visual field for optic nerve meningioma or gliomas.
Check for hearing using 256- and 512-Hz tuning forks.
Look for signs of ataxia and focal weakness.

Consider neuroimaging
Only if history and exam suggest intracranial involvement.
Subependymal nodules are seen with both CT and MRI and are pathognomonic of TS.
"Railroad" calcification of CT or x-ray is seen in SW.
Meningiomas, ependymomas, schwannomas, gliomas, hemangiomas are frequently seen in many neurocutaneous disorders.

Neurocutaneous syndromes
Embryogically, both nervous system and skin arise from ectoderm. It is not surprising that they share the same pathology.

Tuberous sclerosis
Prevalence is approximately 10 per 100,000 people. Most are diagnosed from age 2 to 6.
It can be sporadic or inherited through autosomal dominant pattern.
The genes TSC 1 and TSC 2 are located on chromosome 9p and 16q, respectively. They encode tumor suppressor proteins, mutation of which leads to hamartomas and tumors.
The classic triad is adenoma sebaceum, epilepsy, and mental retardation.

Neurofibromatosis type 1

Prevalence is approximately 40 per 100,000 or one per 2500 live births. Autosomal dominant.

The gene is located on chromosome 17c.

Most findings are on skin: café au lait spots, molluscum fibrosum, and Lisch nodules.

Other systems affected include bone cysts, pathologic fractures (pseudoarthrosis), glial cell nodules in brain and spinal cord, syringomyelia, pheochromocytoma, precocious puberty.

Neurofibromatosis type 2

Is less common than NF1, incidence is approximately one per 30,000 persons. Autosomal dominant. Most diagnoses are made in 20s and 30s.

The gene is located on chromosome 22.

Most findings are central: *bilateral acoustic schwannomas*, meningiomas, ependymomas.

Ten percent of pts with unilateral acoustic schwannoma have NF2.

In younger pts, they may present with early onset cataract called juvenile posterior subcapsular lenticular opacity.

Sturge-Weber syndrome

Incidence is approximately one per 50,000. Inheritance is sporadic.

Disease is caused by hemangiomas in skin, leptomeninges, and brain.

Hemangioma in the skin causes port-wine stain. If located on upper eyelid, buphthalmos and glaucoma may develop due to ↑ vascularity to the area.

The hemangiomas on the leptomeninges and brain give rise to seizures and focal neurologic deficits.

Ataxic telangiectasia

Is rare, approximately one per 100,000 births. Autosomal recessive.

Unlike other neurocutaneous syndromes (phakomatoses), the telangiectasia is not congenital and occurs near eyes at age 3 to 6.

Ataxia is the predominant symptom, starts around age 1, and progressively gets worse as the child gets older.

von Hippel-Lindau disease

Incidence is approximately one per 36,000. Autosomal dominant. Mean age of diagnosis is 26.

Defect is the VHL gene (a tumor suppressor gene) at chromosome 3q.

It is characterized by hemangioblastomas of retina and CNS, plus pheochromocytoma, cysts, and carcinomas of pancreas and kidney.

Symptomatic and supportive treatment

Cryotherapy or laser ablation for skin tumors and angiomas on the face.

Seizures are controlled with anti-epileptic drugs.

Symptomatic intracranial and spinal cord tumors need to be dealt with surgically.

Focal weakness and ataxia may improve with physical and occupational therapies.

Routine ophthalmologic visits may be needed to monitor visual complications from extraocular or intraocular hemangiomas or tumors.

S — Obtain detailed prenatal and perinatal history

Any exposure to drugs, toxins, infections? Any maternal history of diabetes, endocrine disease? Any family history of neurologic disease, previous pregnancy loss, seizures, mental retardation?

Ask about perinatal history including mode of delivery, birth weight, APGAR score, complications such as infection, hyperbilirubinemia, apnea, intraventricular hemorrhage, and prolonged hospital stay.

Obtain detailed developmental history

Including motor, language, and social skill from birth to present.

If the child has previous normal development followed by regression, it is more suggestive of hereditary neurodegenerative disease rather than cerebral palsy (CP).

O — Evaluate mental ability

Intellectual ability can vary from severely retarded to very intelligent. Mental retardation implies more diffuse brain injury.

Assess attention, comprehension, expression, and social interactions.

Note the distribution and degree of motor involvement

Use scale of 0 to 5 to grade strength. "Paresis" is weakness. "Plegia" is complete paralysis.

- Monoplegia or monoparesis: involving one limb.
- Hemiplegia or hemiparesis: involving side of body.
- Diplegia or diparesis: involving both legs predominantly.
- Quadriplegia or quadriparesis: involving all four extremities.

Determine the characteristic of motor impairment

Observe for any abnormal involuntary movements (dyskinesia). Check the tone. Ask and observe pt perform certain tasks.

- Spastic: is the most common type and caused by lesion in the pyramidal system. Look for hyperreflexia, clonus, positive Babinski, and persistent primitive reflexes.
- Dyskinetic: characterized by abnormal tone regulation, postural control, and involuntary movements. It is caused by lesion in the extrapyramidal system (basal ganglia) with most common etiology being kernicterus and severe anoxia.
  - Athetosis: slow, writhing, involuntary movements.
  - Chorea: abrupt, irregular jerky movements.
  - Dystonia: slow rhythmic movements with abnormal posture and tone.
- Hypotonic: tone is decreased but hyperreflexia is present. Usually associated with diffuse brain malformation.
- Ataxic: is the rarest form of CP and is caused by lesion in the cerebellum or its pathways. Look for head, trunk, and limb ataxia. Sitting may be impaired as well as standing and walking with frequent falls. Hands are ataxic with difficulty feeding and writing.
- Mixed: when two or more forms coexist.

Consider lab studies

If hereditary, metabolic, or neurodegenerative disorders are suspected.

Send for routine labs, lactate/pyruvate (for mitochondrial disease), thyroid-stimulating hormone, liver function tests, NH4 (for urea cycle defect), serum/urine amino acids (for inherited metabolic disorders), and chromosome analysis.

Consider brain imaging

Ultrasound, CT, MRI are available options. Ultrasound is good for neonate because of open fontanels, high sensitivity, and no sedation required.

For older children, CT and MRI are preferred. MRI takes long time to perform and may require anesthesia to sedate pt.

Davidoff-Dyke-Masson syndrome is a radiologic diagnosis describing a unilateral hemispheric volume loss/old stroke, thicker skull, bigger frontal sinus and mastoid air cells, and elevation of sphenoid wing and petrous bone. It is often seen in spastic hemiparesis and hemiplegia.

Consider EEG
EEG is helpful in establishing the brain architecture in neonate and infants.

Cerebral Palsy
The official definition of CP is a "term covering a group of *non-progressive*, but often changing, *motor impairment* syndromes secondary to lesions or anomalies of the *brain* arising in the early stages of its development."

Impairment from spinal cord, peripheral nerve, or muscular lesions is not CP.

CP occurs in approximately two per 1000 live birth and affects approximately 1 million people in the U.S.

CP is caused by insult to immature brain starting from prenatal period up to age of 2. The insult can be vascular, hypoxic, infectious, metabolic, toxic, teratogenic, traumatic, genetic, and idiopathic. The insult is a one-time event and does not progress.

CP is classified by the type and pattern of involvement (e.g., spastic hemiparesis, dyskinetic diplegia, spastic quadriplegia).

Rule out treatable causes of pt's symptom
Many times pts are referred to neurologist with wrong diagnosis of CP. Pt may in fact have correctable lesions such as hydrocephalus and treatable metabolic disorders.

Refer pt to early intervention program as soon as possible
Each state has children support services and regional centers that offer excellent physical, occupational, and speech therapies as well as special education programs.

Physical therapy will help with ambulation, stretch spastic muscles, and prevent deformities.

Occupational therapy trains self-help skills and communication on interpersonal interactions.

Less affected school-age children will need education tailored to their intellectual abilities.

Counseling is needed for these children to adapt to the fact that they will always be different from other people. Educated adults with CP are excellent role models to inspire children with CP as well as normal children.

Medical and surgical symptomatic treatments
Spasticity and dystonia can be treated medically and surgically (see chapter on spasticity).

Orthopedic complications such as dislocation, scoliosis, and contractures can be treated by appropriate orthotics or surgery.

G-tube may be needed in children with swallowing difficulty.

Tracheostomy may be needed for in case of recurrent aspiration.

Peripheral Neuroanatomy
Map of dermatomes

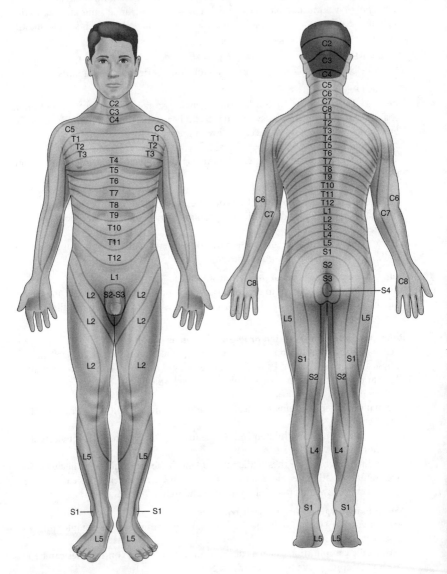

Figure A-1 Dermatome map

Common dermatomes to memorize

Thumb	C5
Little finger	C8
Axilla	T2
Nipple	T4
Umbilicus	T10
Big toe	L5
Little toe	S1
Genital/anus	S1-3

Brachial plexus

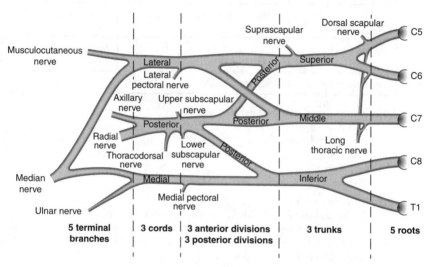

Figure A-2 Brachial plexus

Commonly tested actions, their innervation and nerve roots

Table A-1 Commonly Tested Actions, Their Innervation, and Nerve Roots

Action	Main Muscle(s) Tested	Roots	Peripheral Nerve
Shoulder abduction	Deltoid	C5	Axillary
Elbow flexion	Biceps brachii	C5-C6	Musculocutaneous
Elbow extension	Triceps	C7	Radial
Wrist extension	Extensor carpi radialis and ulnaris	C7	Radial
Finger extension	Extensor digitorum and indicis	C7	Posterior interosseous (deep radial)
Finger flexion (grip)	Hand muscles and flexor digitorum	C8	Median and ulnar
Finger abduction	Dorsal interosseous muscles, abductor pollicis brevis	T1	Ulnar and median

Continued

Table A-1 Continued

Action	Main Muscle(s) Tested	Roots	Peripheral Nerve
Hip flexion	Iliopsoas	L1-L2	Femoral
Knee flexion	Hamstrings	S1	Sciatic
Knee extension	Quadriceps	L3-L4	Sciatic
Ankle dorsiflexion	Tibialis anterior	L4	Deep peroneal (from sciatic)
Ankle plantarflexion	Gastrocnemius, soleus	S1-S2	Tibial (from sciatic)
Foot eversion	Peroneous longus and brevis	L5-S1	Superficial peroneal (from sciatic)
Foot inversion	Posterior tibialis	L4-L5	Tibial (from sciatic)

Important reflexes and their nerve roots

Brachioradialis	C5-C6
Biceps brachii	C5-C6
Triceps	C7-C8
Knee	L2-L3
Ankle	S1

Glasgow Coma Scale

The Glasgow coma scale (GCS) is the scoring system used in quantifying level of consciousness following traumatic brain injury. The scale contains three categories: eye opening (E), motor response (M), and verbal response (V) (Table A-2). The score is the sum of three categories, ranging from 3 to 15.

Table A-2 Glasgow Coma Scale

Eye Opening Response	Best Motor Response	Best Verbal Response
4 spontaneously	6 obeys commands	5 oriented and converse
3 to verbal command	5 localizes to pain	4 disoriented and converse
2 to pain	4 flexion withdrawal	3 inappropriate words
1 no response	3 flexor posturing	2 incomprehensible sounds
	2 extensor posturing	1 no response
	1 no response	

If the patient is intubated, verbal part (V) cannot be assessed and letter "T" is added to the score.
The range will be from 2T to 10T.
A GCS score of 13 to 15 is considered minor injury; 9 to 13 indicates moderate injury; 5 to 8 indicates severe injury, and 3 to 4 indicates very serious injury.

Stroke Syndromes

Some are rare and are listed below only for pimping purpose. They are listed roughly in order of frequency. The typical large vessel strokes (middle, anterior, and posterior) are not included here.

Pure motor
Corona radiata, posterior limb of internal capsule, cerebral peduncle, or ventral pons.
Contralateral weakness.

Pure sensory
Ventral posterior lateral and ventral posterior medial thalamic infarct.
Contralateral sensory loss.

Mixed sensory and motor
Internal capsule and thalamus.
Contralateral hemiparesis and sensory loss.

Ataxic hemiparesis
Basis pontis involving descending corticospinal tract and pontine nuclei.
Contralateral weakness and ataxia.

Dysarthria clumsy hand syndrome
Genu of internal capsule.
Contralateral clumsy hand and dysarthria.

Wallenberg's syndrome (lateral medullary syndrome)
Involves dorsolateral medulla (CN5, CN9, CN10), usually due to posterior inferior cerebellar artery infarct.
Ipsilateral ataxia, Horner's syndrome, ipsilateral facial sensory loss with contralateral limbs loss of pain and temperature.

Weber's syndrome
Ventral midbrain (CN3, cerebral peduncle), due to partial posterior cranial artery infarct.
Ipsilateral CN3 palsy with contralateral limb weakness.

Balint syndrome
Bilateral parietal-occipital stroke.
Simultagnosia, optic ataxia, spatial disorientation.

Gerstmann syndrome
Non-dominant parietal lobe lesion (angular gyrus).
Agraphia, acalculia, right/left confusion, and finger agnosia.

Anton's syndrome
Bilateral occipital infarct.
Denial of blindness, confabulation.

Claude's syndrome
Dorsal midbrain (red nucleus, CN3).
Ipsilateral CN3 palsy and contralateral ataxia/tremor.

Hemiballismus
Subthalamic nucleus.
Contralateral hemiballismus.

Prosopagnosia
Inability to recognize faces.
Bilateral inferior occipito-temporal junction.

Aphasias

Common aphasias
Table A-3 is high yield, but don't try to memorize it. Just understand the points and you can reconstruct the table easily.

Table A-3 Common Aphasias

	Fluency	Comprehension	Repetition
Broca	×	O	×
Wernicke	O	×	×
Conduction	O	O	×
Transcortical motor	×	O	O
Transcortical sensory	O	×	O
Mixed transcortical	×	×	O
Global aphasia	×	×	×

1. Broca's area (inferior frontal gyrus) is required for language output (fluency).
2. Wernicke's area (superior temporal gyrus) is required for language input (comprehension).
3. Arcuate fasciculus (the white matter tract that connects Wernicke's to Broca's area) is required for repetition (in order to be able to repeat, you need to receive the input and transfer it to output center to be articulate).
4. There are higher-level language association areas (sensory and motor) in the brain that work with Wernicke's and Broca's areas to understand and produce language, respectively.

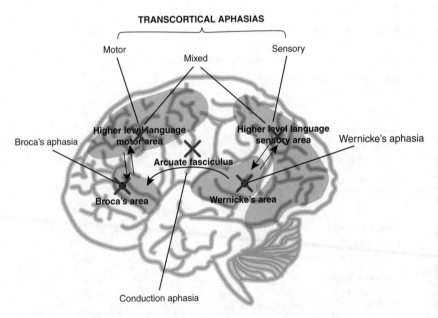

Figure A-3 Common aphasias

Special aphasias

Aphemia
Verbal aphasia without agraphia. Lesion located in small portion of dominant Broca's area or supplement motor area.

Alexia without agraphia
Cannot read but can write. Lesion located in dominant occipital lobe and genu of corpus callosum.

Alexia with agraphia
Auditory comprehension and speech are intact. Lesion located in angular gyrus of dominant parietal lobe. May be part of Gerstmann syndrome.

Pure word deafness
Specific inability to hear spoken language. Other sound perceptions are normal. Lesion located in dominant primary auditory cortex.

Index

A

ABCs, in increased intracranial pressure, 20
Abducent nerve, 2
Abscess, epidural, 65
Absence seizures, 35
Acromegaly, 106
Acute spinal cord syndromes, 64–65
Acyclovir, in herpes simplex virus encephalitis, 51
Adenoma, pituitary, 106
Afferent pupillary defect, 70
Agraphia, 157
Alexia, 157
Altered mental status, 40–41
Alzheimer's disease, 133–134
Amaurosis fugax, 10
Ambulation, 124
Amyotrophic lateral sclerosis, 96–97
Anatomic localization, of disease, 3
Aneurysm
  carotid artery, 73
  saccular, 17
Angiography
  in brain death, 43
  in subarachnoid hemorrhage, 17
Angioma, 23
Anhidrosis, 76
Anterior cord syndrome, 64
Antibiotics
  in bacterial meningitis, 49
  in Lyme disease, 59
  in neurosyphilis, 53
Antibodies, in myasthenia gravis, 83
Anticonvulsants
  in brain injury, 25
  in epilepsy, 30, 31, 37
  in status epilepticus, 33
Antidiuretic hormone, inappropriate secretion of, 25
Antipsychotics, in dementia, 135
Antitoxin, in botulism, 87
Anton's syndrome, 155
Anxiety, 114
Aphasia, 155–157
Aphemia, 157
Apnea, sleep, 140–141
Apnea-hypopnea index, 140
Apneustic respiration, 24

Apraxia, 126, 132
Arbovirus encephalitis, 50
Arnold-Chiari malformation, 19
Arteriovenous malformation, 22, 23
Astrocytoma, 104
Ataxia
  in cerebral palsy, 150
  in Wernicke-Korsakoff syndrome, 44, 45
Ataxia-telangiectasia, 149
Aura
  of migraine, 112
  of seizure, 28
Axonopathy, 89
Azathioprine, in chronic inflammatory demyelinating polyradiculoneuropathy, 91

B

Baclofen pump, 67
Bacterial meningitis, 48–49
Balint syndrome, 155
Becker muscular dystrophy, 94, 95
Bell's palsy, 100–101
Benign occipital epilepsy, 34
Benign paroxysmal positional vertigo, 79
Benign rolandic epilepsy, 34
Benzodiazepines, in status epilepticus, 33
Bilevel positive airway pressure, 141
Biopsy
  muscle, 92, 94, 147
  nerve, 89
Blood pressure, 126
  in hemorrhagic stroke, 9
  in stroke, 7
Blurry vision, 70
Borrelia burgdorferi infection, 58–59
Botterell, Hunt, and Hess scale, 16
Botulinum toxin injection, 67
Botulism, 86–87
Bovine spongiform encephalopathy, 57
Brachial plexus, 153
Bradykinesia, 124
Brain
  herniation of, 20, 21
  injury to, 24–25
  tumors of, 104–105
Brain death, 42–43
Brain scan, 43

Broca's aphasia, 156
Bromocriptine, 106
Brown-Séquard syndrome, 64
Brudzinski sign, 48

C

Café au lait spots, 148
Calcium channel blocker, in subarachnoid hemorrhage, 17
California virus encephalitis, 50
Capillary telangiectasia, 23
Caput medusae, 23
Carbamazepine, 30
 in neuropathic pain, 117
Carbidopa/levodopa, 125
Carotid artery, aneurysm of, 73
Carotid endarterectomy, 11
Carpal tunnel syndrome, 98
Cataplexy, 138, 139
Cavernous malformation, 22–23
Cavernous sinus syndrome, 72–73
Central cord syndrome, 64
Central core disease, 93
Central herniation, 20
Centronuclear myopathy, 93
Cerebellar tremor, 128, 129
Cerebral palsy, 150–151
Cerebral venous thrombosis, 12–13
Cerebrospinal fluid examination. *See* Lumbar puncture
Cherry red spot, 71
Cheyne-Stokes breathing, 24
Children, stroke in, 14–15
Cholinesterase inhibitors, in dementia, 135
Chronic inflammatory demyelinating polyradiculoneuropathy, 90–91
Cingulate herniation, 20
Claude's syndrome, 155
Clostridium botulinum infection, 86–87
Clumsy hand syndrome, 155
Cluster headache, 114–115
Cocaine, 14
Cocaine eye solution, 77
Colloid cyst, 105
Communicating hydrocephalus, 18–19
Computed tomography
 in cavernous sinus syndrome, 72
 in cerebral palsy, 151
 in cerebral venous thrombosis, 13
 in epilepsy syndromes, 34
 in floppy baby syndrome, 145
 in hydrocephalus, 18
 in myasthenia gravis, 83
 in neurocysticercosis, 54
 in opportunistic infections, 60
 in seizure, 28
 in status epilepticus, 32
 in stroke, 6
 in subarachnoid hemorrhage, 16, 17
Concentration, 2
Concussion, 25
Conduction aphasia, 156
Confusion, 40–41
Congenital muscular dystrophy, 95
Consciousness, level of, 2, 154
Continuous positive airway pressure, 141
Contusion, 25
Coordination, 3
Corkscrew sign, 13
Corneal reflex, 42
Corpus callostomy, 35
Cortical sensory function, 3
Corticobasal ganglionic degeneration, 126, 127
Corticosteroids
 in bacterial meningitis, 49
 in Bell's palsy, 101
 in chronic inflammatory demyelinating polyradiculoneuropathy, 91
 in dermatomyositis, 93
 in multiple sclerosis, 121
 in optic neuritis, 71
 in polymyositis, 93
Cough reflex, 42
CPAP, 141
Cranial nerves
 in amyotrophic lateral sclerosis, 96
 in cerebral venous thrombosis, 12
 in diplopia, 74–75
 evaluation of, 2
 in Guillain-Barré syndrome, 84
Craniopharyngioma, 105
Craniotomy, 9
 in increased intracranial pressure, 21
Creutzfeldt-Jakob disease, 56–57
Cryptococcosis, 61
Cushing's response, 24
Cyclophosphamide, in chronic inflammatory demyelinating polyradiculoneuropathy, 91
Cyst, colloid, 105
Cysticercosis, 54–55

D

Dandy-Walker malformation, 19
Davidoff-Dyke-Masson syndrome, 151
Deafness, 78
Decerebrate posture, 24
Dementia, 132–135
   Alzheimer's, 133–134
   frontotemporal, 134
   Lewy body, 126, 127, 134
   secondary, 134–135
   vascular, 134
Demyelinating polyradiculoneuropathy, 90–91
Department of motor vehicles, 29
Depression, 114, 132
Dermatomes, 152–153
Dermatomyositis, 92, 93
Dermoid cyst, 105
Desipramine, in neuropathic pain, 117
Diazepam, in status epilepticus, 33
Diet, ketogenic, 35
Differential diagnosis, 3
Diffuse axonal injury, 25
Digital subtraction angiography, in cerebral venous thrombosis, 13
Diplopia, 74–75
Distal muscular dystrophy, 95
Distal symmetric sensorimotor polyneuropathy, 89
Dix-Hallpike maneuver, 79
Dizziness, 78–79
Doll's eye test, 24
Dopamine agonists, in Parkinson's disease, 125
Doppler ultrasonography
   in brain death, 43
   in subarachnoid hemorrhage, 17
Double vision, 74–75
Driving, 29
Drugs. *See also specific* drugs
   dementia and, 135
   myopathy and, 93
   tremor and, 128
Duchenne muscular dystrophy, 94, 95
Duloxetine, in neuropathic pain, 117
Duret hemorrhages, 20
Dysarthria, 155
Dysequilibrium, 78
Dyskinesia, in cerebral palsy, 150

E

Eastern equine virus encephalitis, 50
Edrophonium test, in myasthenia gravis, 82–83
Electroencephalography
   in altered mental status, 41
   in brain death, 43
   in cerebral palsy, 151
   in Creutzfeldt-Jakob disease, 57
   in dementia, 133
   in epilepsy, 30, 34, 36, 37
   in herpes simplex virus encephalitis, 51
   in peripheral neuropathy, 88
   in seizure, 28
   in status epilepticus, 32, 33
Electromyography
   in amyotrophic lateral sclerosis, 97
   in Bell's palsy, 101
   in chronic inflammatory demyelinating polyradiculoneuropathy, 91
   in entrapment neuropathy, 98
   in floppy baby syndrome, 144
   in Guillain-Barré syndrome, 84
   in mitochondrial disorders, 147
   in myopathy, 92
Electronystagmography, 79
Emery-Dreifuss muscular dystrophy, 95
Empty delta sign, 13
Encephalitis, viral, 50–51
Encephalopathy, Wernicke, 44
Entrapment neuropathy, 98–99
Ependymoma, 104
Epidermoid cyst, 105
Epidural abscess, 65
Epidural hematoma, 25
Epilepsy, 30–31
   frontal lobe, 36
   localization of, 36–37
   occipital lobe, 37
   parietal lobe, 37
   temporal lobe, 36
Epilepsy syndromes, 31, 34–35
Epley maneuver, 79
Erythema migrans, 58
Essential tremor, 128–129
Evoked potential test, in multiple sclerosis, 120
Excessive daytime sleepiness, 138, 139
Extraocular muscles
   in diplopia, 74–75

in Horner syndrome, 76
in myasthenia gravis, 82
Eye
  pain in, 70
  sympathetic innervation of, 76–77

F

Facial nerve, 2
Facial nerve palsy, 100–101
Facioscapulohumeral muscular dystrophy, 95
Familial tremor, 128
Febrile seizures, 35
Floppy baby syndrome, 144–145
Food poisoning, 86–87
Foot drop, 99
Fosphenytoin, in status epilepticus, 33
Freckles, 148
Frontal lobe dysfunction, 132
Frontal lobe epilepsy, 36
Frontal release signs, 126, 133
Frontotemporal dementia, 134
Funduscopic examination, 70–71

G

Gabapentin, 30
  in neuropathic pain, 117
Gag reflex, 42
Gait, 3
  in Creutzfeldt-Jakob disease, 56
  in Parkinson's disease, 124
  in Wernicke-Korsakoff syndrome, 44, 45
Gaze, in diplopia, 74–75
Gaze palsy, 24
Gerstmann syndrome, 155
Glasgow coma scale, 154
Global aphasia, 156
Glossopharyngeal nerve, 2
Glycogen storage diseases, 93
Gower's sign, 94
Guillain-Barré syndrome, 84–85, 90

H

Hallucinations, 138, 139
Headache, 110–111
  cluster, 114–115
  migraine, 112–113
  rebound, 115
  stroke and, 14
  in subarachnoid hemorrhage, 16
  tension, 114–115
Hearing, 78
Hematoma, 25

Hemiballismus, 155
Hemorrhage
  Duret, 20
  intracerebral, 8–9
  subarachnoid, 16–17
Heparin, in cerebral venous thrombosis, 13
Herniation, brain, 20, 21
Herpes simplex virus encephalitis, 50–51
Horizontal gaze palsy, 24
Horner syndrome, 76–77
Human immunodeficiency virus (HIV) infection, 61
Huntington's disease, 133
Hydrocephalus, 18–19
Hydrocephalus ex-vacuo, 19
Hydroxyamphetamine solution, 77
Hypercoagulability state, stroke and, 13, 14
Hyperthyroidism, in myasthenia gravis, 82
Hypnagogic hallucinations, 138, 139
Hypoglossal nerve, 2
Hypokalemic periodic paralysis, 93
Hypothermia, 42
Hypothyroidism, in myasthenia gravis, 82
Hypotonia, 144–145
  in cerebral palsy, 150

I

Immune globulin
  in chronic inflammatory demyelinating polyradiculoneuropathy, 91
  in Guillain-Barré syndrome, 85
Inclusion body myositis, 92–93
Infant
  botulism in, 87
  hypotonic, 144–145
Infarction, spinal, 65
Infection
  in cerebral venous thrombosis, 12
  meningeal, 48–49
  viral, 50–51, 61
Infectious polymyositis, 93
Inflammatory demyelinating polyradiculoneuropathy, 90–91
Insomnia, 141
Intention tremor, 129
Internuclear ophthalmoplegia, 75
Intracerebral hemorrhage, 8–9
Intracranial pressure
  in hemorrhagic stroke, 8–9
  increase in, 18–19, 20–21
  normal, 20
Ischemic stroke, 6–7

J

Juvenile myoclonic epilepsy, 35

K

Kearns-Sayre syndrome, 147
Kernig sign, 48
Kernohan's notch, 20

L

La Crosse virus encephalitis, 50
Laceration, brain, 25
Lambert-Eaton syndrome, 83
Lamotrigine, 30
Landau Kleffner syndrome, 35
Lateral medullary syndrome, 155
Leigh disease, 147
Lennox Gastaut syndrome, 34–35
Levetiracetam, 30
Lewy body, 125
Lewy body dementia, 126, 127, 134
Lidocaine, in neuropathic pain, 117
Light, pupillary reaction to, 75
Limb-girdle muscular dystrophy, 95
Lipoma, 105
Lobectomy, in epilepsy, 37
Lorazepam, in status epilepticus, 33
Lumbar puncture
   in bacterial meningitis, 48
   in chronic inflammatory demyelinating polyradiculoneuropathy, 91
   in Creutzfeldt-Jakob disease, 56–57
   in Guillain-Barré syndrome, 84
   in headache, 111
   in herpes simplex virus encephalitis, 50
   in hydrocephalus, 18
   in Lyme disease, 58–59
   in multiple sclerosis, 120
   in neurocysticercosis, 54
   in neurosyphilis, 53
   in opportunistic infections, 60
   in optic neuritis, 71
   in peripheral neuropathy, 89
   in seizure, 28
   in status epilepticus, 32
   in subarachnoid hemorrhage, 16–17
Lyme disease, 58–59

M

Mad cow disease, 57
Magnetic resonance imaging
   in acute spinal cord syndromes, 65
   in amyotrophic lateral sclerosis, 97
   in cavernous sinus syndrome, 72
   in cerebral palsy, 151
   in cerebral venous thrombosis, 13
   in Creutzfeldt-Jakob disease, 57
   in dementia, 133
   in entrapment neuropathy, 98
   in epilepsy, 30, 34, 36
   in floppy baby syndrome, 145
   in herpes encephalitis, 50
   in hydrocephalus, 18
   in mitochondrial disorders, 147
   in multiple sclerosis, 120
   in neurocysticercosis, 54
   in opportunistic infections, 60
   in optic neuritis, 71
   in seizure, 28
   in stroke, 6
   in subarachnoid hemorrhage, 17
   in vertigo, 79
Mannitol, in increased intracranial pressure, 21
Mechanical ventilation, 141
Medulloblastoma, 105
MELAS (myopathy, encephalopathy, lactic acidosis, and strokes), 147
Memory, 2
   loss of, 132
Meningioma, 105
Meningitis
   bacterial, 48–49
   viral, 51
Mental status, 2
   altered, 40–41
   in amyotrophic lateral sclerosis, 96
   in cerebral venous thrombosis, 12
   in Creutzfeldt-Jakob disease, 56
   in dementia, 132
   in ischemic stroke, 6
   in Parkinson's disease, 124
   in Wernicke-Korsakoff syndrome, 44
Meralgia paresthetica, 99
MERRF (myoclonic epilepsy with ragged red fibers), 147
Midazolam, in status epilepticus, 33
Migraine, 112–113
   stroke and, 14
Miller-Fisher syndrome, 85
Miosis, 76
Mitochondrial disorders, 146–147
Mixed transcortical aphasia, 156
Monro-Kellie doctrine, 20

Motor examination, 2–3, 153–154
  in acute spinal cord syndromes, 64
  in amyotrophic lateral sclerosis, 96
  in cerebral palsy, 150
  in chronic inflammatory demyelinating polyradiculoneuropathy, 90
  in Guillain-Barré syndrome, 84
  in muscular dystrophy, 94
  in myasthenia gravis, 82
  in peripheral neuropathy, 88
Motor neuron disease, 96–97
Multiple sclerosis, 71, 120–121
Multiple system atrophy, 126, 127
Muscle biopsy, 92, 94, 147
Muscle spasm, 66–67
Muscular dystrophy, 94–95
Myasthenia gravis, 82–83
Myelinopathy, 89
Myelitis, transverse, 65
Myoclonic epilepsy with ragged red fibers (MERRF), 147
Myoclonus, in Creutzfeldt-Jakob disease, 56
Myopathy, 92–93
  in floppy baby syndrome, 145
Myopathy, encephalopathy, lactic acidosis, and strokes (MELAS), 147
Myositis, 92–93
Myotonia, 94
Myotonic dystrophy, 94–95

N

Narcolepsy, 138–139
NARP (neuropathy, ataxia, and retinitis pigmentosa), 147
Nausea, 78
Neck, stiffness of, 24
Nemaline myopathy, 93
Nerve biopsy, 89
Nerve conduction study
  in amyotrophic lateral sclerosis, 97
  in Bell's palsy, 101
  in botulism, 87
  in chronic inflammatory demyelinating polyradiculoneuropathy, 91
  in entrapment neuropathy, 98
  in floppy baby syndrome, 144
  in Guillain-Barré syndrome, 84
  in mitochondrial disorders, 147
  in myopathy, 92
  in peripheral neuropathy, 88
Neuritis, optic, 70–71
Neurocutaneous syndromes, 148–149
Neurocysticercosis, 54–55
Neurofibromatosis, 148, 149
Neurogenic shock, 24
Neurologic examination, 2–3
  in altered mental status, 40
  in bacterial meningitis, 48
  in botulism, 86
  in brain injury, 24
  in brain tumor, 104
  in cavernous sinus syndrome, 72
  in cluster headache, 114
  in diplopia, 75
  in epilepsy, 30
  in headache, 111
  in Horner syndrome, 76
  in Lyme disease, 58
  in migraine, 112
  in mitochondrial disorders, 146
  in multiple sclerosis, 120
  in myopathy, 92
  in neurocysticercosis, 54
  in neuropathic pain, 116
  in neurosyphilis, 52
  in opportunistic infections, 60–61
  in seizure, 28
  in sleep apnea, 140
  in spasticity, 66
  in status epilepticus, 32
  in subarachnoid hemorrhage, 16
  in vascular malformation, 22
  in vertigo and dizziness, 78
Neurologic history, 2
Neuronopathy, 89
Neuropathic pain, 116–117
Neuropathy, 88–89
  entrapment, 98–99
  in floppy baby syndrome, 144, 145
  optic, 71
  peroneal, 99
  ulnar, 99
  in Wernicke-Korsakoff syndrome, 44
Neuropathy, ataxia, and retinitis pigmentosa (NARP), 147
Neuropsychological testing, in dementia, 133
Neurosyphilis, 14, 52–53
Non-communicating hydrocephalus, 18–19
Normal pressure hydrocephalus, 18, 19
Nortriptyline, in neuropathic pain, 117
Numbness
  in Guillain-Barré syndrome, 84
  in stroke, 6
Nystagmus, 44, 56, 78

O

Obstructive sleep apnea, 140–141
Occipital lobe epilepsy, 37
Ocular palsy, 74–75
Oculocephalic reflex, 42
Oculomotor nerve, 2
Oculopharyngeal muscular dystrophy, 95
Olfactory nerve, 2
Oligodendroglioma, 104
Olivopontocerebellar atrophy, 127
Ophthalmoplegia, 44
Opioids, in neuropathic pain, 117
Opportunistic infections, 60–61
Optic nerve, 2
Optic neuritis, 70–71
Optic neuropathy, 71
Oral contraceptives, stroke and, 14
Orientation, 2
Otorrhea, 24
Oxcarbazepine, 30

P

Pain
  eye, 70
  head. See Headache
  neuropathic, 116–117
Palsy, Bell's, 100–101
Papilledema, 75
Papillitis, 70
Parietal lobe epilepsy, 37
Parkinson plus syndromes, 126–127
Parkinsonism, 132
Parkinson's disease, 124–125
Paroxysmal hemicrania, 115
Periodic lateralizing epileptic discharges, 51
Periodic limb movement disorder, 141
Periodic paralysis, 93
Peripheral neuropathy. See Neuropathy
Peroneal neuropathy, 99
Phenobarbital, 30
  in status epilepticus, 33
Phenytoin, 30
  in status epilepticus, 33
Pick's disease, 134
Pituitary gland, tumors of, 106–107
Plasmapheresis
  in chronic inflammatory demyelinating polyradiculoneuropathy, 91
  in Guillain-Barré syndrome, 85
Polymyositis, 92, 93
Polyradiculoneuropathy, demyelinating, 90–91
Polysomnography, 140
Port-wine stain, 148
Posterior cord syndrome, 64
Posture, in Parkinson's disease, 124
Pregnancy, stroke and, 14
Presyncope, 78
Primitive neuroectodermal tumor, 104
Prions, 57
Progressive external ophthalmoplegia, 147
Progressive multifocal encephalitis, 61
Progressive supranuclear palsy, 127
Prolactinoma, 106
Propofol, in status epilepticus, 33
Proprioception, 3
Prosopagnosia, 155
Proximal symmetric sensorimotor polyneuropathy, 89
Psammoma bodies, 105
Pseudodementia, 132
Psychosis, Korsakoff, 44
Ptosis, 76
Pupil
  afferent defect of, 70
  examination of, 75
  light reaction of, 42, 86
Pure word deafness, 157

R

Ragged red fibers, myoclonic epilepsy with, 147
Rapid plasma reagin (RPR), 52
Reflex(es), 154
  corneal, 42
  cough, 42
  in dementia, 133
  gag, 42
  oculocephalic, 42
  in Parkinson plus syndromes, 126
  pupillary, 42, 86
Reflex epilepsy, 35
Residual ischemic neurologic deficit, 10
Respiration
  apneustic, 24
  Cheyne-Stokes, 24
  in Guillain-Barré syndrome, 84
Restless leg syndrome, 141
Rhinorrhea, 24
Rhizotomy, 67
Rigidity, 124
Riluzole, 97
Romberg test, 44
Rubral tremor, 129

S

St. Louis virus encephalitis, 50
Scotoma, 70
Seizure, 28–29
  absence, 35
  febrile, 35
Senile tremor, 128
Sensory examination, 3
  in acute spinal cord syndromes, 64–65
  in chronic inflammatory demyelinating polyradiculoneuropathy, 90
  in peripheral neuropathy, 88
Shagreen patches, 148
Shock, neurogenic, 24
Shunt, in hydrocephalus, 19
Shy-Drager syndrome, 127
Sleep
  hygiene for, 139
  stages of, 139
Sleep apnea, 140–141
Sleep paralysis, 138, 139
Somatosensory evoked potentials, in brain death, 43
Spasticity, 66–67
Speech, 2
Spinal accessory nerve, 2
Spinal cord syndromes, 64–65
Stalk section effect, 106
Status epilepticus, 32–33
Striatonigral degeneration, 127
Stroke, 154–155
  anterior, 7
  brainstem, 6
  cerebellar, 6
  in children, 14–15
  cocaine and, 14
  cortical, 6, 7
  hemorrhagic, 8–9
  ischemic, 6–7
  migraine and, 14
  oral contraceptives and, 14
  posterior, 7
  pregnancy and, 14
  subcortical, 7
  syphilis and, 14
  transient ischemic attack and, 11
  in young adults, 14–15
Sturge-Weber syndrome, 148, 149
Subarachnoid hemorrhage, 16–17
Subdural hematoma, 25
Subfalcine herniation, 20
Superior orbital fissure syndrome, 73

Syndrome of inappropriate antidiuretic hormone secretion, 25
Syphilis, 52–53

T

Tabes dorsalis, 52
Taenia solium infection, 54–55
Tarsal tunnel syndrome, 99
Taste sensation, 100
Tay-Sachs disease, 148
Telangiectasia, capillary, 23
Temporal lobe epilepsy, 36
Temporal lobectomy, 31
Tensilon test, in myasthenia gravis, 82–83
Tension headache, 114–115
Thiamine
  deficiency of, 44–45
  intravenous, 45
Thrombolytic therapy, in stroke, 7
Thrombosis, venous, 12–13
Thymectomy, in myasthenia gravis, 83
Thymoma, in myasthenia gravis, 83
Tinel test, 98
Tissue plasminogen activator, in stroke, 7
Titubation, 129
Todd's paralysis, 28, 32, 54
Tolosa Hunt syndrome, 73
Tonsillar herniation, 20
Topiramate, 30
Touch, 3
Toxoplasmosis, 60–61
Tramadol, in neuropathic pain, 117
Transcortical motor aphasia, 156
Transcortical sensory aphasia, 156
Transcranial Doppler ultrasonography
  in brain death, 43
  in subarachnoid hemorrhage, 17
Transient ischemic attacks, 10–11
Transverse myelitis, 65
Trauma, brain, 24–25
Tremor
  essential, 128–129
  in Parkinson's disease, 124
Trigeminal nerve, 2
Trochlear nerve, 2
Tuberculosis, 61
Tuberous sclerosis, 148
Tumors
  brain, 104–105
  pituitary, 106–107
Two-point discrimination, 3

U

Uhthoff phenomenon, 70
Ulnar neuropathy, 99
Ultrasonography
　in brain death, 43
　in subarachnoid hemorrhage, 17
Uncal herniation, 20
Uvulopalatopharyngoplasty, 141

V

Vagus nerve, 2
Vagus nerve stimulator, 31
Valproic acid, 30
　in status epilepticus, 33
Vascular dementia, 134
Vascular malformation, 22–23
Venereal Disease Research Laboratories (VDRL) test, 52
Venezuelan equine virus encephalitis, 50
Venous malformation, 23
Venous thrombosis, 12–13
Ventilation, mechanical, 141
Ventriculoatrial shunt, 19
Ventriculoperitoneal shunt, 19
Ventriculostomy, in increased intracranial pressure, 21
Vertigo, 78–79
Vestibular nerve, 2
Vibration, 3
Vigabatrin, 30
Viral encephalitis, 50–51
Viral meningitis, 51
Vision, double, 74–75
Visual field, 70
Visual-spatial function, 2, 132, 133
Vital capacity, in Guillain-Barré syndrome, 84
VITAMINS mnemonic, 40–41
Vomiting, 78
Von Hippel-Lindau disease, 149

W

Wada test, 31, 37
Wallenberg's syndrome, 155
Warfarin, in cerebral venous thrombosis, 13
Weakness
　in Guillain-Barré syndrome, 84
　in stroke, 6
Weber's syndrome, 155
Wernicke-Korsakoff syndrome, 44–45
Wernicke's aphasia, 156
West Nile virus encephalitis, 50
Western equine virus encephalitis, 50
Word deafness, 157
Wound botulism, 87
Wrist drop, 99

X

Xanthochromia, in subarachnoid hemorrhage, 17

Z

Zonisamide, 30